DATE DUE

NOV 2 6 1995		
APR - 1 1997		
MAR 1 2 1991		
APR - 2 1998		
APR 1 0 1998		
APR 2 3 2008		
SEP 1 0 2008		
GAYLORD .		PRINTED IN U.S.A.

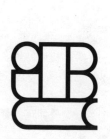

COLLABORATIVE MANAGEMENT IN HEALTH CARE

MARTIN P. CHARNS AND

LAURA J. SMITH TEWKSBURY

COLLABORATIVE
MANAGEMENT
IN
HEALTH CARE

Implementing
the
Integrative
Organization

Jossey-Bass Publishers · San Francisco

For sales outside the United States, contact Maxwell Macmillan International Publishing Group, 866 Third Avenue, New York, New York 10022.

Manufactured in the United States of America

Library of Congress Cataloging-in-Publication Data

Charns, Martin P., date.
  Collaborative management in health care : implementing the integrative organization / Martin P. Charns and Laura J. Smith Tewksbury.
      p.   cm.—(A joint publication in the Jossey-Bass health series and the Jossey-Bass management series)
  Includes bibliographical references and index.
  ISBN 1-55542-483-X
  1. Health services administration. 2. Health services administration—Case studies. 3. Organizational change.
  4. Organizational change—Case studies. I. Smith Tewksbury, Laura J., date. II. Title. III. Series.
RA971.C517   1993
362.1′068—dc20   92-26467
                                                                CIP

FIRST EDITION
HB Printing   10 9 8 7 6 5 4 3 2 1   *Code 9283*

A joint publication in

The Jossey-Bass

Health Series
and
The Jossey-Bass

Management Series

To my wife, Judy,
and my mom, Edna

To my parents
and my brother;
to my husband, Robert,
and my son, Griffin

Contents

Preface

The 1980s was a decade of both unprecedented turmoil and advancements in health care, and the 1990s are bringing even greater challenges and changes. Old paradigms of management are being discarded and new ones are being developed. Most health care managers and clinicians have realized that their organizations are not truly responsive to patients, but they may not be able to see how they can make significant improvements. Although many remedies have been tried, little progress has been made toward reversing the fragmentation of care and of management.

In most health care organizations, the professional disciplines function as if they were a series of vertical chimneys, with patients bouncing from one chimney to the next over the course of care. Each discipline tends to have its own perspective on patient care and to function fairly autonomously. Management efforts also have historically been highly fragmented, with clinicians and administrators often working at cross-purposes, communicating ineffectively, and blaming each other for the problems in their organization and in health care in general. Often, individuals' extraordinary efforts save the day, as everyone works around highly dysfunctional structures, systems, and procedures. People tend to blame problems on other departments, but too often they simply have no effective way to resolve those problems. Many decisions are based more on protecting power and turf than on anything else. Individual disciplines have taken on greater importance than patients, notwithstanding the rhetoric in statements of missions and goals. As the parts have become more important than the whole, both patients and staff have suffered the consequences.

We believe that a major reason for the problems in health care is that traditional organizational structures hinder both delivery of care and effective management and fragment efforts rather than facilitate them. Until the mid 1980s, most health care managers accepted the basic structure of their organizations as unchangeable and did not think about how structure affects the behavior of employees or staff. Nor did they understand how to design and implement new structures effectively. Thus, although health care managers have made some changes in management practices, they have been limited by traditional hierarchical structures that promote fragmentation. And when structural changes have been attempted, they have often been unsuccessful, creating new problems as bad as or worse than the old.

One organizational approach that often (but not always) included structural change was product line management, which became popular in health care in the mid to late 1980s. It had the potential to reduce fragmentation but was poorly defined and poorly understood. Much of the literature about it was highly prescriptive, but the advice of different authors conflicted. Some institutions claimed to have succeeded with product line management, but the number of failures reported eventually tarnished the concept.

It was at that time and in that environment that this book was conceived. We saw that although health care organizations had access to many concepts through organizational literature, managers were not applying them effectively. To address the clear need for change in the industry and to provide guidance to managers and clinical leaders who want to improve their organizations, we developed a framework based on organization design. That framework is presented through a continuum of organizational configurations.

Although we began our work with a review of the product line management literature and practice, we saw more flexible ways of working with organization design. Thus, we chose to focus on *integrative approaches* to management and delivery of care. As part of our research, we studied a variety of sites and developed six original case studies. The results of that detailed work, as well as our experience in teaching and consulting, highlighted the importance of structure but also revealed other critical factors. Those included the selection of people to serve in key integrative positions, support for the new structure through reward and information systems, and the process of implementing change.

Who Should Read This Book?

This book was written for health care executives and clinical leaders who want to improve the functioning of their organizations. The general framework we offer and the specific examples we analyze can provide guidance in designing and implementing organizational innovations to improve productivity, quality of work life, and responsiveness to the needs of patients and their families. We also illuminate the many pitfalls and unintended dysfunctional outcomes that lie along the way and offer advice about how to avoid them.

We have clarified and defined terms that are often misused, in an effort to provide a common language for clinicians and managers to use in discussing organizational issues. Thus *Collaborative Management in Health Care* can also be helpful in disseminating ideas about organizational innovation and helping people understand the change process. The book also will be useful to students of health care management in graduate and continuing education programs in schools of management, public health, nursing, medicine, and other health professions.

Organization of the Book

The book is organized into two parts. The conceptual framework is presented and developed in Part One. In addition to the theory, we have included numerous short examples of the concepts as well as suggestions for their use. In Chapter One, we discuss the special characteristics of health care that affect efforts to improve the industry, and we explain our framework for organization design and change. Nine basic organization structures are analyzed in Chapter Two, and each is placed on a continuum of organization design choices. The characteristics, pros, and cons of each choice are described in detail.

Effective organization design is inextricably related to the characteristics and skills of members as well as leaders of an organization. When an organization is undergoing structural change, the selection of managers who will see the effort through is crucial to success. Chapter Three addresses management challenges in integrative organizations as well as criteria for choosing managers and determining what skills they should have. It also discusses several alternatives for combining integrative responsibilities with traditional professional roles.

Chapter Four explains both formal and informal rewards and the importance of instituting a reward system that supports— and does not undermine or inhibit—the desired new behaviors and the change process. New types of information are needed to attain the benefits of an integrative structure, and Chapter Five discusses information requirements from a nontechnical perspective. In addition, since many health care organizations have implemented new information systems without updating their structures, Chapter Five also examines the organizational requirements for using sophisticated information systems to aid in decision making. Chapter Six identifies the critical factors that can determine whether an organizational change will succeed or fail. Through concepts and examples, we highlight potential pitfalls in orchestrating a change process and ways to avoid them.

Having established a conceptual framework for understanding integrative management, in Chapter Seven we look at product line management as a special case. The chapter reviews the literature on this approach and clarifies the objectives of putting product line management into effect. We reconcile conflicting recommendations in the literature by matching the different possible objectives of product line management with the organizational alternatives presented in Chapter Two.

Because health care organizations are so complex and multifaceted, and because success in organizational innovation depends on many factors, readers gain both knowledge and insight through actual examples of the concepts in practice. Therefore, in Part Two, we present six detailed case studies of health care institutions in the process of change. Each case study addresses conceptual issues, notes specific characteristics of the teaching or community hospital in question that assist or hinder integrative management, and demonstrates the benefits, limitations, and pitfalls of the organizational structure and the change process. Each case is rich in detail. Chapters Eight through Thirteen each focus on a single case. The case studies are presented in order, according to the degree of integration of their structures and where they fall on the organizational continuum presented in Chapter Two.

Although the cases are based on actual situations, the names, locations, and specific details have been thoroughly altered. The names of staff and employees, the names of neighboring institutions, landmarks, and the like, have all been fabricated to lend the cases verisimilitude while completely obscuring the actual identities of the institutions we studied.

The cases illustrate both successes and failures of organizational innovation in a variety of settings and organizational types. Two are university teaching hospitals, two are community hospitals, and two are community hospitals with some teaching programs. Four are single, freestanding hospitals, one is a two-campus hospital formed through a merger, and one is a three-hospital operation in the process of being merged.

In the concluding chapter, we reflect on the conceptual framework, the interrelationships among organization design, selection of integrative managers, rewards and information systems, and change process, and how they are exemplified in the case studies. We then place the framework in perspective among the many actions effective leaders must take to implement innovative, responsive organizations.

Acknowledgments

People at the six organizations that are the subjects of the case studies gave us their time, access to confidential and critical information, and honest opinions about the successes and failures of change efforts at their institutions. The cases are highly disguised because we did not want to be limited in our analyses of their experiences or hold back criticism that could assist others. We thank the leaders and members of these organizations for participating in our research, and we commend them for their pioneering efforts, even though not all were successful.

We thank our colleagues at Boston University and Concord Hospital for their support and constructive criticisms, and for granting us the time to work on this project. Just Stoelwinder provided valuable feedback as we were formulating our conceptual framework, and he has been a continual source of intellectual stimulation and support. Arnold Kaluzny and anonymous reviewers also provided many helpful suggestions on the manuscript.

Our research for and preparation of *Collaborative Management in Health Care* have spanned nearly four years. During that time, one of the authors was married, and both became parents. We have spent many days away from home and countless hours at our word processors. For their support and patience we deeply thank our spouses, Judy and Robert.

We hope that our efforts will inspire new paradigms for organizing to meet the challenges the health care industry faces as we enter the twenty-first century.

August 1992   Martin P. Charns
                                               Newton, Massachusetts

                                               Laura J. Smith Tewksbury
                                               Concord, New Hampshire

The Authors

Martin P. Charns is president of Associates in Health Care Management, Boston-based international management and organizational consultants. He has been on the faculty at the Boston University Schools of Public Health and Management, and teaches in the Program for Chiefs of Clinical Services at the Harvard University School of Public Health.

Charns received his B.S. degree (1967) from Case Institute of Technology in mathematics and his M.B.A. degree (1969) from Harvard University, where he was a Baker Scholar. Continuing studies at Harvard, he began research on health care organizations and received a D.B.A. degree (1972). He was assistant professor of organizational behavior at the Graduate School of Industrial Administration at Carnegie-Mellon University, and associate professor of organizational behavior and health care management at Boston University School of Management. He managed the executive education programs in health care management and served as director *ad interim* of the Health Care Management Program.

Charns is coauthor (with M. J. Schaefer) of *Health Care Organizations: A Model for Management,* selected by *Hospitals* as one of the best management books of 1984. He has published numerous articles and more than fifty case studies. He has twenty years' consulting experience, has worked with organizations in many industries and in government, and has specialized in health care.

Charns was chairman of the Health Care Administration Division of the Academy of Management (1987–1988) and is a member of the National Advisory Committee for Strengthening Hospital Nursing: A Program to Improve Patient Care, jointly sponsored by the Robert Wood Johnson Foundation and the Pew Charitable Trusts. He is a member of the editorial board of *Medical Care Review* and is a reviewer for the *Journal of Hospital and Health Services Administration* and the *Journal of Health Administration Education.*

Laura J. Smith Tewksbury received her B.S. degree (1980) from the University of New Hampshire in health administration and planning and her M.B.A. degree (1989) from Boston University with a concentration in health care management.

Tewksbury has worked in health care planning and management for twelve years, through a progression of staff and line management positions. She has conducted extensive research into the planning and implementation of product line management in hospitals and was responsible for putting service line management into place in a community hospital setting.

She is the author of two related articles: "Product Line Management and Continuum of Care," and "From Product Line to Service Line: Health Care Adopts Successful Business Technique to Reduce Costs."

COLLABORATIVE MANAGEMENT IN HEALTH CARE

PART ONE

Effective Organization

Design and Change

The first part of this book presents the conceptual framework for health care organization design and implementation of change. It begins, in Chapter One, with the challenges facing health care and the premises on which the framework is built. The organizational continuum, which is the organizing framework for the book, is presented in Chapter Two. Nine prototypical organizational forms are presented, and the strengths and limitations of each are discussed. In Chapter Three the selection of integrative managers, their skills, influence, and reporting relationships are examined. Specific attention is given to the different personnel requirements needed to operate the different structures. Chapter Four addresses rewards, considering both formal extrinsic rewards and rewards potentially available from work itself. Chapter Five discusses information systems, information requirements, and the congruence between an organization structure and information system. In Chapter Six, concepts and techniques for implementing organization change are discussed. Although the concepts have wide application, special

1

attention is given to implementing integrative structures. Product line management is the topic of Chapter Seven, where we view it from the perspective of the organizational continuum and discuss its strengths and limitations.

Chapter One

The Challenges
of Improving
Organization
Effectiveness

This is a book about making health care organizations more effective—more responsible to patients, more timely and efficient in delivering services, more satisfying for professional staff, and more collaborative in relations with physicians. This is a tall order. Yet, a review of the organization design and management literature—together with research, consultation, and discussion with numerous health care managers—leads us to conclude that most health care organizations could perform much more effectively than they currently do.

Many efforts have been made to improve the functioning of hospitals in recent years. Although the federal government has changed hospital regulations and incentives, the continuing public outcry over the health care system indicates that results have not been altogether satisfactory. Costs have continued to rise. Access to care has been limited, and quality has been questioned. Managers in many hospitals, sometimes in response to these pressures, have tried a variety of interventions aimed at improving staff satisfaction and care delivery. These have included training programs, quality

circles, employee incentive programs, financial bonuses, staff surveys, information systems, team building, management retreats, collaborative practice, cross-training of workers, product line management, organization restructuring, and, most recently, total quality
management (TQM) and continuous quality improvement (CQI).

Virtually all work organizations are complex, and hospitals
are among the most complex of organizations. Therefore, an approach that is sufficient to make substantial, lasting, positive
changes in hospital functioning must take into account the multifaceted character of hospitals and address issues in a systemwide
manner. None of the approaches to organizational improvement
that we have just mentioned can be used in isolation to achieve the
level of organizational performance needed. Other concepts and
skills are needed to manage an organization effectively.

It is striking to us that few approaches to hospital improvement place much emphasis on the design of organization structure.
Most do not consider it at all. Yet the organization design of most
hospitals and other health care organizations hinders the achievement of both clinical and management work. Through the personal
efforts of dedicated professionals who are concerned for patients, the
organizations achieve their current levels of performance in spite of
their organization design. In fact, whether planned or not, most
health care organizations are structured more for the professional
disciplines than for the patients, notwithstanding the organizations' stated patient care goals. Analyses of health care organizations based on Stoelwinder and Charns's Task Field Model of
Organization Analysis and Design (1981) support this opinion.
Most health care professionals with whom we have worked reach
this same conclusion once they are given a conceptual framework
that allows them to critique their organizations.

Only a few years ago, it would not have been possible to cite
many examples of major structural changes in hospitals directly
affecting delivery of care. Although many hospitals had developed
corporate forms of organization, the purpose was to allow the hospitals to garner income from for-profit activities without affecting
their nonprofit status. Consequently, the core of the organization
involved in the delivery of care was not directly affected. Similarly,
hospitals have shifted accountability for departments from one vice

president or assistant administrator to another, significantly affecting the distribution of power, but not having any substantial impact on the interaction among caregivers or the actual delivery of care. In contrast, in response to environmental change and turbulence, as well as to increased competition, greater financial pressures, work force shortages, and the desires to be more responsive to patients and have better relations with physicians, a small but growing number of health care organizations have now implemented a variety of new organization designs and management systems.

Although the examples of both successes and failures we present in this book are drawn from our research and consultation in the United States, we have directly participated in implementing similar organization changes in hospitals in Australia and Canada, and have observed like efforts in Great Britain. The imperative for improving health care delivery and experimentation with organization design are global phenomena; they are not unique to the United States but are characteristic of countries with very different systems for financing and paying for health care.

Efforts at health care reorganization typically have gone under the rubric of product line management, service line management, matrix organization, or strategic business units. Some of these represented major changes in organization structure. However, they have had varying degrees of success in terms of affecting the behavior of staff and attaining stated objectives. In some organizations the efforts appear to have been motivated by a desire to follow a fad, often adapting approaches that have worked in other industries. While some of these attempts have been successful in health care, others have not only failed to attain the desired results, they have generated ill will. Many organization change efforts, both within the United States and around the world, have lacked the structure of a valid conceptual framework. This book aims to provide such a framework, thereby, we hope, contributing to both theory development and practice.

Goals of This Book

The main goal of this book is to illustrate how work in health care organizations can be coordinated better and how problems can be addressed and solved more effectively. We describe a conceptual framework for organizational diagnosis, and offer guidance in the selection and implementation of organization structures and systems. We also provide examples, in the form of detailed case studies, of ways to apply the conceptual framework successfully.

The framework we offer is primarily one of organization design, that is, the arrangement of people, work, and responsibilities. The design of an organization has an important influence on what happens, how people interact, what work is done, and what is not done. Health care managers can use organization design as a management tool. However, to be used effectively, organization design needs to be combined with other approaches to organization change. For example, we have successfully used organization design together with CQI, multidisciplinary collaborative practice, case management, and the implementation of multiskilled workers. In doing so, we have relied on many organization development techniques, such as management retreats, team building, and responsibility charting. Probably the most important point we can make in setting the context for this book is that organization design is a powerful tool that is underutilized as a vehicle for health care organization improvement, but one that should not be used in isolation.

In most industries, organization design is reflected in the formal authority structure. In health care, however, physicians generally are not employees of the organization, and consequently are not subject to the same rewards and sanctions as employees are. This book provides a broadened view of organization theory that allows for its effective application to health care in light of the special involvement of physicians. This is important, for, as the case studies will illustrate, inadequate physician involvement has been at the root of many failures in organizational innovation.

Premises

Our framework is built on the following five key premises:

1. The design of the structure of an organization substantially affects organizational performance. Good people make a difference; but consistent, strong organizational performance cannot be achieved only *by recruiting good people. To manage individual behavior without managing organization structure and systems is to work at a disadvantage.*

Central to effective organization design is facilitating collaboration among people whose work dictates that they work interdependently (Charns and Schaefer, 1983, pp. 123-124). Often in health care, the organization structure actually hinders effective work relationships. This is true in the performance of both clinical and management work. The structure, professional training, rewards and incentives, information system, and culture all reinforce independent efforts rather than collaboration. Many administrative and clinical professionals in health care function as if their part is more important than the whole. The model of a health care organization made up of independent entrepreneurs and fiefdoms may have been feasible when reimbursement was cost based and the prevailing premise was that the professional alone knew what was best for the patient. Now, in a time characterized by strong patient rights and desire for involvement, competition, and increased attention to both cost and quality of care, such a model is no longer viable.

As we explain in Chapter Two, most health care organizations reflect the basic "functional" organization form common at the turn of the century. Our observation is that political forces and maintenance of the rights and responsibilities of each profession and specialty have contributed to the perpetuation of this organization form. While the flow of patient care has not deliberately been given a lower priority than professional development, one effect of the functional structure is support for individual professions and hindrance of the flow of care.

Maintenance of the traditional structure may stem from the beliefs of both clinical and management professionals that good people make a good organization, and that good people can work in any structure. We agree that good people are critically important to a successful organization, but we disagree with the belief that structure is not important.

Also contributing to the persistence of the status quo is the belief of many hospital executives that they should not interfere in the clinical aspects of their organization and that they do not control the medical staff organization. Although these beliefs are changing, many non-clinically trained managers are reluctant to initiate change that directly affects clinical workers. Medical practitioners in leadership positions also often resist administrative incursions into what they see as their areas of responsibility.

Not all organizations truly are "designed," as we are using the term. Instead, they typically evolve in response to multiple competing forces. Nonetheless, whether managers or clinicians are aware of it or not, and whether any particular structure has actually resulted from a design process, structure is always working to influence what information people receive, how it is reported and interpreted, what relationships develop among people and what loyalties they have, and the priorities they give to requests from others. In this way, structure directly affects an organization's ability to recognize, analyze, and solve problems. In fact, structure not only affects how well people work together to solve problems, but also what issues people identify as problems worthy of their attention and efforts.

For example, in most traditionally structured hospitals, no one department assumes "ownership" of a patient throughout the whole course of care. Each department "owns" a patient only while it provides its particular service or procedure. This contributes to the fragmentation of care, which is exhibited in many different situations. One such situation arises when a patient needs to be transferred from one part of the hospital to another. Concerned about their own work load and the increased demands that accompany the arrival of a new patient, staff on a unit that is to receive a patient try to delay the transfer. Concerned exclusively about their own work load, the staff transferring the patient want to relieve themselves of the responsibility as soon as possible. Typically, neither group has information about what is happening in the other department. Their information, and therefore their focus, concerns only their own demands. Furthermore, a department rarely ever receives information on overall patient outcomes or satisfaction. Therefore, staff virtually never have either the perspective or the responsibility for the total patient experience. A frequent result is a tug of war, or a negotiation, between the two groups, with each trying to present its situation to the other in a light that will give it the advantage.

A similar pattern emerges when patients are discharged. The nursing staff may not let Admitting know that a bed is available, thereby deferring an increase in their work load that would result from a new admission. Admitting's goals are to utilize beds as soon as they become available and get patients into rooms rather than hold them in Admitting or the Emergency Department. Staff in any given unit are focused on caring for patients currently under their aegis, balancing their work load, delivering services as well as possible to their patients. A patient waiting for a bed is not "their" patient. They do not have to confront the actual condition of that patient or his or her need to get to the unit. If they had information about the individual, they might alter their actions to facilitate the admission. But without the information, the incoming patient is not part of their perceived reality. Similarly, the staff in Admitting, not specifically aware of the complexity, dynamics, and work load on the unit, cannot fully appreciate or take into account the situation there. They may push to place a patient on a unit that is not clinically appropriate for that person or push for a more rapid response from the unit than they are able to provide. Important here is that each workgroup acts on its own limited pool of information and is focused narrowly, rather than globally, in the organization. There are many other possible examples of ways structure affects information flow—and, therefore, behavior. These effects can be positive and assist good people, or they can be negative and cause good people to expend extreme amounts of energy to accomplish good work in spite of the organization.

Health care organizations are placing greater emphasis on marketing and on relations with medical staff and patients. Often these efforts are attempts to shift the organizational focus from inputs to the care process (that is, the contributions of the various departments) to outputs (the total care provided for patients). Organizations vary in their conceptualizations of outputs, with definitions based on diagnosis-related groups (DRGs), major diagnostic categories, clinical services, patients of particular groups of physicians, or market segments. We have observed, however, that in health care organizations where substantial structural changes are being implemented, managers and clinicians rarely have a sound understanding of the overall effects of organization design or of the tradeoffs inherent in their newly adopted structure.

2. Coordination of work affects performance, and it is fool-hardy to leave coordination of critical activities to chance.

Coordination and organization structure go hand in hand. Structure always facilitates coordination of some work and people and it always hinders coordination of other work and people. When work is not coordinated, its quality and its timeliness suffer. This is a basic law of organization. We can ill afford either low quality or lack of timely delivery of services.

Well-managed organizations put structures and processes in place to ensure coordination. Coordination, like quality, cannot be added after services are delivered. It must be built into the delivery of service. It also must be built into management decision-making and problem-solving structures (such as task forces and committees), systems (such as information and evaluation systems), and processes (such as how staff actually interact). In order to achieve coordination, however, each discipline must truly place its self-interest second to the interests of patients and the organization.

3. Rewards and information affect individual and organizational performance, and one of the most powerful sources of reward and information is the work itself.

We know from the discipline of psychology that rewards affect individual behavior. Unfortunately, we often forget to apply that knowledge in managing organizations of all types, including health care. Too often we reward one particular behavior, when we really hope people will behave in a different way (Kerr, 1975). For example, we reward individual departments for their success in competing against each other for budget, space, and other scarce resources within an organization, yet we hope that they will cooperate in the best interests of the organization as a whole. Some organizations punish departments that do not spend all of their allotted resources by reducing their budgets in subsequent years, at the same time hoping that managers will spend responsibly.

Most health care workers have chosen their field because of the nature of the work itself and the inherent rewards it offers. Thus the potential for motivation is great. Unfortunately, we often frustrate these people, making it difficult or impossible for them to do their work effectively. In so doing, we deprive them of the rewards inherent in doing their work well. Not only do we eliminate the most powerful source of motivation, we also burn out many of our most talented professionals—the ones who really care.

Rewards affect all types of behavior. In one state-owned teaching hospital, whose support services were particularly unresponsive, staff were very frustrated by their inability to get the services their patients needed. The staff often dealt with this frustration by being absent from work, but few ever quit their jobs. Moreover, it was difficult to recruit new staff. Professionals in the community as well as in the hospital knew it was not a rewarding place to work. Yet, the rewards for staying—among them employee benefits and a vested state retirement plan—deterred the staff from leaving the hospital, even after they lost their motivation to work hard.

Performance feedback is another major factor in people's behavior. What people hear and what they do not hear may have important but opposite effects. When people hear relevant feedback about their performance on the job, they generally alter their behavior. Relevant performance feedback is generally both reinforcing and motivating to the people who receive it. When feedback is uneven and addresses only some aspects of performance, individuals may respond solely to that information, missing the larger issues and changing their behavior in inappropriate ways. Examples of this are plentiful in organizations. Feedback based solely on volume of service, for example, risks encouraging people to sacrifice quality. Feedback limited to patient satisfaction may risk undermining employees' attention to cost. Feedback on only the short-term effects of people's actions encourages them to focus on short-term success, with less concern for long-term implications. Similarly, feedback on departmental performance that excludes overall organizational performance encourages people to focus on their own departments, which contributes to interdepartmental conflict.

Good information is critical to effective management. Information is the essential ingredient in decision making and in problem solving. Most health care organizations, however, do not collect or disseminate information on program performance. Rather, health care information systems were developed as financial reporting systems, to relate the organization's financial performance to the public and to obtain reimbursement for services provided. Since reimbursement historically has been based on aggregate costs, it is aggregate data that have been collected and reported. Furthermore, the aggregation has followed the lines of the internal organization structure, so information on the fiscal performance of individual departments and cost centers is all that has been available to managers of the typical hospital.

The prospective payment system has been a major force in redefining hospital information needs. Initiated by the federal government for medicare patients and adopted by other payers, the prospective payment system pays a hospital a fixed amount for each type of case, or diagnosis-related group (DRG), regardless of actual costs. This has reduced hospitals' abilities to pass their costs on to government and insurers, thereby increasing hospitals' need to contain costs. To manage costs of different types of cases, hospital managers must have departments' cost information broken down by case type, or DRG.

In addition, competition and other financial pressures have given rise to hospital managers' need for information on costs, revenues, volumes, and profitability, broken down not only by diagnosis and DRG but also by physician, specialty, and patient source. When such detailed information is provided to physicians, in a form that compares their resource use and length of stay to those of others, it can increase each physician's understanding of his or her impact on the financial health of the hospital. This can raise physicians' motivation to give more attention to resource utilization.

The high performance standards in innovative hospitals demand that more information in more accessible forms be available in multiple, diverse locations. Such hospitals require, for example, obtaining as much patient information as possible prior to admission; minimizing the burden, inconvenience, and repetition of information collection; facilitating the delivery of patient information to physicians, whether in the hospital, office, home, automobile, or elsewhere; and monitoring actual interventions and patient progress against expected progress, so that needs for clinical or managerial interventions can be determined and so that the timing of related services (such as arranging for postdischarge care) can be anticipated and planned for.

Even when a hospital's organization structure facilitates delivery of care with responsiveness to patients and physicians, that structure is still limited by the information available and the capabilities of the information system. Conversely, the impact of a sophisticated information system is limited by an organization's ability to use that information—a factor that is greatly affected by its structure. Many health care organizations are expending significant sums of money for systems that provide management and clinical information in forms useful for program decision making. However, if the organization is structured so that responsibilities for programs are diffused, information cannot be used effectively. Furthermore, clinicians and managers cannot be expected to use a new information system effectively immediately after it is implemented. As with any sophisticated tool, the use and application of an information system must be learned, with skills developing over time.

Addressing these issues requires more than a technical solution that makes additional information available. When people receive too much information, they selectively limit what they perceive and act upon. Thus, although there is no simple answer to the problem of information management, there are better and worse ways of handling it. The implications of these issues and their relation to the organization's structure and information system will be discussed throughout the book.

4. The systems and approaches that are best for one organization are not necessarily best for another, even within the same industry; they should be designed to address the unique environment, mission, and strategy of each specific organization.

Organization theory has moved well beyond the belief that any one organizational form is universally best. Instead, it is widely agreed that form should follow function, that is, that organization design should follow organization strategy. Unfortunately, too often we see organizations copy another's approach without analyzing it adequately—and then wonder why it did not work for them. Organizations are unique in their environments, strategies, work forces, resources, strengths, and weaknesses, as well as in their cultures and histories. All of these factors need to be considered in choosing an organization's best approach to a wide array of organizational and management issues, and, indeed, in simply determining what approaches it is possible for any given organization to implement.

Adapting approaches from other industries may provide valuable ideas, because substantial organizational experimentation and innovation have occurred outside of health care. However, not all factors or assumptions on which others' approaches are based will apply equally well or in the same way in health care. Many factors even differ from one hospital to another. Thus, an organization adapting the structure of another must recognize and understand the critical similarities and differences between the two organizations.

5. Management work is different from clinical work. To be performed effectively, management work requires mastery of management skills and concepts.

Many very smart people have discovered the hard way that general intelligence does not take the place of learning the skills that are needed to manage an organization effectively. As an analogy, consider a passenger riding in an airplane many times and expecting that experience to be an adequate foundation for flying it. Performing clinical work in a hospital does not equip a person with all of the skills and concepts that are needed to manage the organization effectively. Both organizational and managerial skills and knowledge are required, as well as interpersonal skills. Perhaps out of frustration, some physicians and other clinical professionals have assumed that they can manage their health care organizations better than their current administrators, and that success in their own profession presupposes their ability to be good managers. Experience has shown this not to be true. Some people learn management through formal training; others, through experience, the guidance of a competent mentor, and a program of personal reading. Either way, learning the applicable concepts and developing the necessary skills makes success much more likely than "winging it."

The Uniqueness of Health Care

The histories of most health care organizations have been marked by strained relations among their key groups of personnel. The hospital's formal authority structure has often been described as a "three-legged stool," consisting of trustees, administration, and medical staff. Overt strains also are commonly seen among administration, nursing, and the medical staff, although "turf battles" extend to other health professions and also exist among medical specialties. Yet, the need for cooperation in decision making is as critical among these groups in health care as it is among any groups in any kind of organization.

Many factors have worked to divide administrators, nurses, and physicians. Historically, they have been trained in different schools, used different theoretical frameworks, and employed different "languages." They have been influenced by different professional literatures and organizations, and have been legally authorized to perform different tasks. The functions they learn to perform result in very different approaches to problem solving, with different time horizons, expectations, and patience for results. Although their overall aim is the same—quality, cost-effective care—the three have been responsible for different aspects of providing health care services, with individual goals that are inherently conflicting. They have tended to work independently, without directly interfering in each other's spheres of responsibility. In reality, the trio consisting of administrator, nurse, and physician needs to be expanded to include the many ancillary and support departments that play major roles in the effective provision of quality care. In an episode of care, a patient may easily encounter special services ranging from dietary to rehabilitative therapy to social work, with each department playing a key role in the care of the patient and having a need for a collaborative relationship with the other care givers.

This separation of professionals is problematical for effective management of health care organizations. Too many clinical and managerial decisions require the groups to work together to plan, to diagnose problems, and to implement plans and solutions. Given the history in some organizations, however, requiring a member of one group to report to a member of another group raises hackles. Even suggesting that the groups work collaboratively sometimes generates resistance. Furthermore, even willing parties often are difficult to get together because of the logistics of their different work and schedules. Thus, the professions operate within what look like separate "vertical chimneys" in the organization, with little or no assistance in crossing over from one to another. This provides a challenge to implementing innovative organizational forms. As we will describe, some organizations have addressed this challenge effectively, while others have not.

The Need for Consistent Terminology

In health care organizations, difficulties often arise merely through the lack of common terminology. Not only do separate "languages" make collaboration difficult among different disciplines, they are also impediments to the use of concepts from organization and management literature with clinical professionals. Not knowing the technical definition of the term *functional organization*, someone not trained in organization and management might simply believe it means "an operation in which the structure works"; in other words, one that is "functional" rather than "dysfunctional." Ironically, however, a functional organization can be dysfunctional with respect to the effective delivery of care. The definition is, simply, an organizational form in which the major units in the organization represent professional and nonprofessional *functions* (Charns and Schaefer, 1983). *Matrix organization* and *team* are also terms that have different meanings for different people. In addition, some terms, such as *committee*, may be weighted with connotations, such as inefficiency and unproductive time, that cloud their objective meanings.

Other terms are used in different ways in different contexts. For example, *department* is often used to refer to organizational units such as the Nursing Department, Social Service Department,

Housekeeping Department, Admitting Department, and so on. However, *department* may also refer to the Department of Medicine, Department of Surgery, Department of Pediatrics, and the like. These are also often called services. *Services* may also refer to the range of diagnostic and therapeutic procedures offered by a facility or to the care delivered to patients. More specifically, it can refer to the activities of the Social Services Department. The term *unit* can refer not only to the generic "organizational unit," which is any aggregation of people in an organization's hierarchy, but also to a "patient care unit" or "nursing unit." Many people use the terms *patient care unit* and *nursing unit* interchangeably. Other people use *nursing unit* to imply that the space and the people working there are part of the Department of Nursing. This implies that others who see patients there are not a central part of the unit. These different uses of the term have implications for how people behave and for their commitment to making the unit work effectively.

Throughout this book, we take special care to explain terms and work to avoid ambiguities. We ask the reader to be alert for multiple meanings of terms, both in this book and in practice. Until a more consistent terminology is accepted widely, there is great risk for miscommunication.

Organizational Innovation

Some new organizational forms and systems implemented over the last several years by health care organizations might simply be called "changes," whereas others are "innovations." Distinguishing characteristics of innovative hospitals are their new standards for effective management of patients and for facilitating relationships with physicians. These new standards place a central emphasis on service, responsiveness to patients and physicians, effective utilization of resources, and management of individual cases to utilize patients' time in the hospital as effectively as possible. Thus, in deciding what to call an innovation, we have chosen to focus on organization changes that affect its basic way of delivering service. We have consciously excluded superficial changes, such as customer relations programs, that may do no more than add a smile to a poorly delivered service. We have chosen to focus on integration and decision making because these are so critical to an organization's functioning and success.

In health care, integrative organization structures represent relatively uncharted territory, with few organizations having tried to implement anything very different from tradition and fewer still being systematically studied. Some have turned to the broader management and organization literatures for guidance. We believe this is a good place to start, but it is not enough, for it does not reflect health care's differences in mission, goals, environment, work force, culture, and history, as compared to other industries.

Conceptual Framework

Two major themes in the organization and management literature have particular relevance for health care. The first is integrating the diverse elements of a health care organization to provide continuity—rather than fragmentation—of both patient care and management. All too often, health care decision making resembles the well-known tale of the six blind men and the elephant. Each person believes that his or her limited perspective constitutes the "truth," when only together can they recognize that the parts they bring to the process make up a greater whole. In the tale, each of six blind men touches a different part of an elephant and argues from his perspective that the elephant is actually a wall (side), a spear (tusk), a snake (trunk), a tree (leg), a fan (ear), and a rope (tail). Of course they all are incorrect, owing to their limited perspectives (Saxe, 1970).

The second management theme of special use to health care is the sharing of decision-making responsibility and authority, and the placing of these as close as possible to the sources of relevant information in the organization, rather than requiring information and decisions to travel through layers of hierarchy. This requires empowerment of middle- and supervisory-level managers. It also requires allowing and empowering people at different levels and with different responsibilities—not only line managers but staff as well—to take the lead and the responsibility for solving problems and implementing efforts that cross into others' areas of responsibility. Many issues in complex health care organizations cut across formal lines of authority; yet it is rare for managers to take the lead in addressing these issues and, when they do, to receive cooperation from managers of areas they cross into. It is not surprising that this is difficult in traditional organizations, for crossing into others' areas of responsibility runs counter to traditional management teachings and is seen as an "intrusion," in most organizational cultures. It is often interpreted as a threat by department managers who see it as a challenge to their power and control. Thus, substantial effort is required to allow, encourage, and support efforts that cross organizational lines of authority.

To address these complex issues, this book presents a framework built on the concepts of organization design. The first premise of the framework is that a carefully chosen organization design can balance an organization's need for different types of coordination and its need to specialize in its various parts. Further, the framework considers organization design a vehicle for carrying out organizational strategy, although it will not address how to choose that strategy. Also, the framework addresses the critical factors in selecting personnel to fill integrative positions in hospitals, and the effective use of reward, management control, and information systems. Since how a change is introduced and implemented can be as important to its success as making the right choice of structure, people, or systems, the book examines key factors in managing change.

Chapter Two

The Continuum of Organization Structures

An organization's structure has an important influence on the outlook and behavior of people who work in the organization. Yet, this topic has received relatively little attention in the health services literature. In this chapter we will discuss the theory behind organization design and review prototypical organizational forms. Although it is unusual to find an organization that is a pure prototype, knowledge of the characteristics of the prototypical forms provides a solid basis for understanding the variations. Each organizational form has inherent strengths and weaknesses. Each addresses some organizational needs well and hinders attainment of others. The art of organization design is in the selection of a structure and set of systems that best suit a given organization's requirements.

Structural Contingency Theory

The guiding theoretical framework for this book, structural contingency theory, was initially developed in the for-profit business sector. In contrast to earlier theories, which sought a way of organizing that was applicable to all organizations, contingency theory is built on the premise that an organization's structure, systems, and practices should be designed to meet the unique requirements of its task and environment (Woodward, 1965; Thompson, 1967; Lawrence and Lorsch, 1967). Although in retrospect this does not seem to be such a radical concept, it represented a major break with previous theories. Galbraith (1973) built upon the work of earlier contingency theorists, conceptualizing organizations as information processing systems. Galbraith's characterization of how organizations increase their information processing capacity through the addition of various structures, processes, and other mechanisms provided the basis for our development of the framework presented in this chapter.

Few organizationwide applications of structural contingency theory to health services organizations can be found in the literature. Most published articles describe an application in one organization, typically focusing exclusively on the advantages of the approach presented. These works generally provide neither a conceptual base for the approach nor adequate detail to determine its appropriateness for other situations. When they refer to organizational types, such as "matrix" organizations, they often use the terminology inaccurately and apply the concepts incorrectly.

Papers that describe measurement of organizational characteristics also typically have been limited to one or, occasionally, a small number of sites. However, they usually have been driven by a conceptual framework that allows generalization. Fottler (1987), in his review of research on health care organizational performance, notes that "most of the studies concerned with [structural determinants of performance] use only *one* dependent variable. Consequently, it is difficult to determine what structural types or organizational characteristics contribute the most to *overall* performance because we usually only have performance along one dimension" (p. 374). Empirical studies need to be organizationwide if they are to constitute true research on organization design, but few meet this criterion. It is costly to collect in-depth, organizationwide data. Therefore, studies tend to be limited in depth, rigor, and/or sample size.

One of the first empirical applications of structural contingency theory to health care was an analysis of eight academic medical centers (Charns, Lawrence, and Weisbord, 1978; Weisbord, 1976). Others include Stoelwinder and Clayton's (1978) intervention in developing ward teams in an Australian hospital; Weisbord, Stoelwinder, and Pava's (1983) involvement of medical staff in decisions to contain costs; Smith and others' (1989) study of physician involvement through a team structure on patient care units; and Harmon and Kirkman-Liff's (1984) review of management teams in a state public health department. McDaniel and others (1987) describe the detail of a decision-making process for organization design applied to a community hospital.

Burns's (1989) research on the evolution of matrix organizations in hospitals differs from the other empirical studies. Its strengths are its large sample size and use of a longitudinal research design. However, it exemplifies the common difficulty of applying theories developed in other industries to health care. A lack of understanding of hospital organization is apparent in the attempt to measure features of matrix structures by analyzing the unit manager position. Managers and researchers familiar with hospitals that have implemented unit management systems are aware that the position is inherently limited by its low level in the hierarchy, lack of authority over any other professional staff, lack of control over resources that could provide a base of power, and tendency to be staffed by personnel who do not carry personal influence in the organization. It is not surprising, therefore, that Burns found little relationship between unit management systems in 1981 and further evolution of matrix organization characteristics in 1987.

Several conceptual articles and book chapters are also worth noting for their contributions to development of organization design in health care. Stoelwinder and Charns (1981) develop the concept of task fields in their analysis of design conflicts that stem from multiple goals of a teaching hospital. Charns and Schaefer (1983) present an organization design framework based on the analysis of clinical and management work. Leatt, Shortell, and Kimberly (1988) also present a comprehensive description of organization design in health care. However, a gap remains between the need for guidance in health care organization design and the available concepts. We intend to address this gap.

Organizational Requirements

Two primary organizational requirements presented in contingency theory are *differentiation* and *integration* (Lawrence and Lorsch, 1967). *Differentiation* refers to specializing parts of an organization to meet the unique requirements of the work performed by each part. In most industries, organizations typically differentiate by functions. In health services, these functions represent the various professions and nonprofessional specialties. Examples are nursing, social work, physical therapy, housekeeping, and admitting. Each function develops goals and internal departmental structures, policies, procedures, and personnel and management practices individually suited to the function.

People within a functional department (the different functional groups typically are called "departments") generally interact with each other more than with people in other departments. Furthermore, much of their conversation concerns the activities of their department. The frequent interactions among people within each department reinforce the goals and interpersonal orientations particular to the function. People in each functional department become a part of the social group of the department, and the group becomes a strong influence on their behavior. Since evaluations are performed by supervisors within a department, and behaviors are rewarded or sanctioned formally through management practices and informally through group interactions, individuals' identifications with their functional department are reinforced. Typically, people look for career advancement within their functional department. This is particularly so in the health professions, where professional identity is critically important. Since in health care the professions most often coincide with the functional departments, professional identity amplifies differentiation by function.

Differentiation is essential to organizational performance. It allows each unique type of work to be performed most effectively. It also provides an organization with links to its environment. In health care, for example, the nursing department typically maintains contact with nursing organizations and imports information on the state of the art in the profession. The nursing department also serves as the representative of the nursing profession within the organization. In that role it works to maintain the profession's standards. Similarly, the housekeeping department, being focused on environmental services, typically provides the organization with information on the state of the art in technique, product, and practice in its area. Housekeeping, for example, has the organizational expertise not only in cleaning techniques but also in handling hazardous materials. A department maintains expert knowledge by having members of the department attend conferences, shows, or seminars, or by having vendors call on the department. In addition to exchanging information, each department serves an important role in attracting and developing personnel specialized to its function. Thus, each differentiated department serves as an organization's "window" on a part of its relevant world. Different departments provide different "windows," each directed at the specialized part of the environment associated with the function.

Integration, or coordination, is also essential to organizational performance. In any complex organization, the work of different individuals and of different parts of the organization is interdependent. This interdependence results from (1) interconnections among the elements of work performed by the different people or parts of the organization, and (2) the need to share resources among people or organizational units. In either case, but especially where interdependence results from the work itself, ineffective coordination can directly reduce the quality and efficiency of work performance. As health services organizations have sought to be more responsive to their consumers and to be more efficient, the importance of effective coordination has increased.

Organizing to facilitate coordination is a central theme in the literature on organization design (see, for example, Thompson, 1967; Lawrence and Lorsch, 1967; Galbraith, 1973). Charns and Schaefer (1983) have summarized this literature and applied it to the design of health care organizations. They note that "one should group people, work and responsibilities so that group boundaries do not break across work interconnections. The organization design should attempt to capture interconnections within the boundaries of any one work group. Where that is not possible, groups responsible for interconnected work should be placed as close as possible to each other in the organization. The reason for this is quite straightforward. Having interconnected pieces of work located in separate parts of the organization makes it difficult to manage the whole, for each unit owns its part more than it owns the whole" (p. 123). Thus, within each organizational unit, coordination among members of the unit is facilitated by patterns of interaction and by common goals, rewards, cognitive and interpersonal orientations, and supervision. It is between units that coordination is most difficult to achieve. This is because differentiation and integration are antithetical, and organizing to achieve one complicates achievement of the other.

The traditional health services organization, with each different department representing a different function, emphasizes *differentiation by function* at the cost of *coordination of functions*. Thus, the performance of each function is optimized independently, and the major difficulties arise in coordinating work and sharing resources among functions. These difficulties can occur in critical areas, however, such as in delivering patient care, which typically requires the efforts of multiple functions. In one community hospital, for example, we noted that seventeen different departments plus medical staff had substantial responsibilities in providing services for a typical patient.

In generalizing these concepts from the functional form to other organizational forms, the same principles hold. Whatever constitutes the basis for determining what each part of an organization represents will be reinforced at the expense of coordination among those parts. Thus, if a health care organization is designed around the different clinical programs it offers, differentiation of programs can be optimized and integration of programs will be problematic. Each program can be designed and managed in the manner most appropriate for accomplishing that program's unique work. However, if patients need to be served by two or more programs or if resources such as staff, space, supplies, or equipment need to be shared among programs, the coordination will present a challenge to the organization. Inherent in the task of achieving integration among the programs is managing the conflict among them.

Hospitals refer fairly consistently to groupings of staff by common discipline or function as "departments." Organizations structured into functional departments are referred to as "functional organizations." There is, however, no consistency in use of terminology for other bases of organizing in health care. In the broader organizational literature, the terms *product division* and *program division* are used to refer to multifunctional units that manufacture products or deliver services, respectively. Product divisions and program divisions are often simply called "divisions." Use of the term *division* in health care in curs a risk of misinterpretation because the term also refers to clinical divisions within medical departments (for example, the division of cardiology within the department of medicine). This can be especially confusing in academic medical centers, where the terms apply both to a medical school and to one or more hospitals. By using the phrase *program division,* we hope to minimize possible misinterpretation. We refer to organizations structured into program divisions as "program organizations."

Programs can represent many different things. Each possible basis for constituting a program facilitates the organization's relationships with a different group or segment of its environment. One basis is groups of patients, such as children, older adults, and women. Organizing along these lines allows a hospital to tailor its services most directly to its different patient groups. Alternatively, a hospital could organize along the lines of the services it offers, such as sports medicine, occupational health, emergency services, and rehabilitation services. This basis of organization allows a hospital to optimize the delivery of each service. Any patient or group of patients may require more than one type of service, however, and coordinating these services is hindered by selecting this basis for organizing. Similarly, a hospital could be structured into programs according to patient conditions, problems, or diagnoses. Examples are cancer, heart problems, and substance abuse. Finally, an organization might use a structure that corresponds to medical specialties or to groups of related specialties. For example, one program that is often found when this basis for design is employed is a neurosciences program, which includes neurology, neurosurgery, and sometimes psychiatry. By organizing according to specialties, a hospital can address relationships with medical staff most directly, but this basis for determining programs may not correspond to client needs very well. Organizing by aggregations of specialties has the advantage of coordinating the specialties within each program. Whichever structure is chosen, coordination among staff within each program will be enhanced and coordination between programs will be hindered.

It is important to clarify one other issue of terminology before proceeding. We have suggested the general term *program* to refer to an integrated set of patient care services delivered to a targeted, possibly uniquely identified, set of clients. Some organizations use the terms *products, product lines, services, service lines, care programs, businesses, centers of excellence,* or *strategic business units.* Each of these has specific connotations, some of which are negative and some of which are misleading. For example, most clinicians do not like to refer to "products" of a health care organization because the term connotes dehumanization and assembly line manufacturing. Also, some people associate a particular set of organization and management practices with each of these terms. To minimize unintended connotations, we will use the term "program" in a general way, to apply to any of the bases of organization we have described. This is consistent with use of the term in many service (in contrast to manufacturing) organizations, such as universities. The term does have other uses in health care—for example, "residency programs," which are not necessarily interdepartmental. The meaning of the term will generally be clear from the context, but we encourage the reader to be alert to the many uses of this term in order to avoid misunderstanding.

Thus far we have discussed organizing either by function or by program, as if the only choices were either entirely one way or entirely the other. However, the two can be used together to address both differentiation and integration, and their various combinations form a continuum.

The Organization Design Continuum

Health services organizations have begun to experiment with innovative designs, and nine prototypical forms represent the major variations. The functional organization and the program organization are opposites in their effects on facilitating differentiation and integration, and as such, they form two ends of a continuum of organization designs. The continuum of organizational structural configurations ranges from a pure functional organization to a pure program organization (see Figure 2.1).

The different structural forms along the continuum represent varying degrees of trade-off between the differentiated functional and integrated program orientations. From left to right on the continuum, the structures provide increasing emphasis on integration (lower portion of rectangle increases from left to right) and decreasing emphasis on differentiation by function (upper portion of rectangle decreases from left to right). At the extreme left end of the continuum, there is nearly total focus on the individual professional and nonprofessional functions and no attention to integration of functions into programs. At the extreme right end of the continuum, the opposite is the case, with emphasis placed on integration of functions within program divisions and little attention to the needs of individual functions. The right end of the continuum represents a complete differentiation by programs, with indi-

Figure 2.1. Continuum of Organizational Configurations.

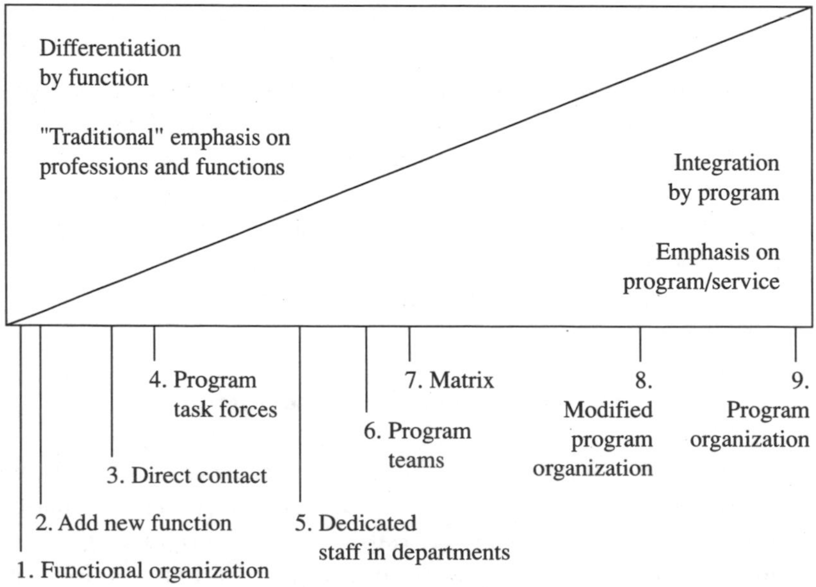

vidual program orientations being reinforced and no integration across program divisions. At the right end of the continuum, the program divisions operate as autonomous businesses, each containing all of the functions it needs. (For additional discussion of organizational structure, refer to Galbraith, 1973, and for applications to health care, refer to Charns and Schaefer, 1983, and Leatt and others, 1988.)

Functional Organization

In a pure functional organization (at the extreme left end of the continuum), responsibilities are divided by function, with the major organizational units in a hospital being departments that represent the different professional and nonprofessional functions (see Figure 2.2). This traditional structure was found in nearly all hospitals until the 1980s and still characterizes many facilities. The functional organization maximizes differentiation and emphasizes management of and professional focus on each function or profession independently. The structure itself provides for no integration of functions to achieve coordinated, comprehensive care, and it affords no managerial focus on programs or other outputs of the hospital that require combined efforts of functions.

Among the functional organization's strengths are the following: allowing economies of scale by pooling and sharing resources within each function; encouraging focus on cost and quality of each functional department's services, which represent inputs to the care process; and maintaining professional competence and contributing to professional development by facilitating peer interaction, and by providing performance review, professional

Figure 2.2. Functional Organization, Simplified Schematic.

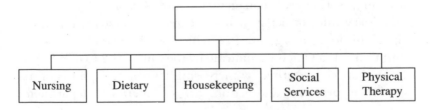

supervision, and support within each department (Charns and
Schaefer, 1983; Stoelwinder and Charns, 1981; Charns and Smith,
1989).

Management focus is placed on each department separately,
and attention is devoted to achieving high performance in each
department individually. In addition, through the frequent interaction among members of each department, the department's goals
and members' commitment to the department are reinforced. Each
department serves as the advocate for the function or profession it
represents; by having all the practitioners of a given profession
within one department, the ability to advocate for the profession is
maximized. In addition, by having a direct reporting relationship
from individual staff through a professional supervisory structure
to senior department management, the department management
has the responsibility and authority to maintain professional standards throughout the organization. For example, the chief nursing
officer can access formal lines of authority to maintain standards of
professional practice and to enforce organizationwide policies.

Weaknesses of the functional structure include encouraging
focus on each department's processes independently, allowing territorialism by function and profession, and, thus, contributing to
fragmentation of care. Furthermore, this structure works against
development of even informal patterns of interaction among personnel from different departments who are interdependent in the
provision of services. Without such consistent relationships, coordination of services is difficult to achieve.

Parallel Organizations

To compensate for the inherent limitations of a functional organization and/or to add new capabilities in areas such as planning,
marketing, or financial management, some hospitals have implemented new roles or departments. There are five structural variations of this form of organization, which we shall call "parallel organization," and which we indicate by the numbers 2 to 6 in Figure
2.1. They are characterized by increasingly greater emphasis on integration of decisions and actions across functional departments

and by increasing capability to manage and coordinate the efforts of the functional departments.

Addition of a New Function

In the first of these parallel organizational forms (number 2 in Figure 2.1), one or more departments, consisting of specialists in areas such as marketing, planning, or finance, are added "parallel" to or alongside the other departments in a functional organization. These functions, which may be new to the organization, represent professional technologies and/or skills, just as nursing, social services, and housekeeping do. Typically, they have organizationwide responsibility for marketing, planning, or financial analysis. From time to time, their efforts may focus on a particular program, patient population, medical specialty, or clinical area—but that temporary focus does not imply continuing responsibility. For example, the planning department in a hospital typically would have the primary responsibility for determining the need for and costs of providing a new service, but its responsibility would be limited to planning and not extend to implementation. Typically, departments concerned with marketing, planning, and financial analysis are viewed as "staff" rather than "line."

A distinguishing characteristic of this form of parallel organization is that the specialists are not given responsibilities for any particular programs. Rather, the hospital remains functionally structured, with one or more new functions, but with the inherent characteristics, strengths, and weaknesses of a functional organization. It does, however, have the additional capabilities of the new function or functions, which may assist slightly in integration across departments. Many hospitals, in fact, have this organizational form but do not consider it a vehicle for facilitating integration across functions. It is questionable on technical grounds whether this structure actually is anything other than a functional organization. The structural form is determined by how the direct work of the hospital is organized. "Staff" work, such as finance, personnel, and security, does not affect the term we use to name the structural form. We have distinguished form 2 from a pure functional form (1) in order to discuss its relative advantages and lim-

itations in providing integration. Its position on the continuum—
very close to 1—indicates its limited integrating capacity.

Direct Contact

In the second form of parallel organization (number 3 in Figure 2.1),
individuals are given responsibility for specific programs. These individuals, whom we shall call "integrative managers" or "program
managers," may be marketing, planning, or finance specialists. Alternatively, they may be managers or clinicians who have other responsibilities and who assume integrative responsibilities. However,
as in all forms of parallel organization, integrative managers do not
have formal authority that spans departments, and functioning of
the organization does not depend on these managers' having direct
supervisory relationships over personnel whose efforts contribute to
their programs. They must rely on their interpersonal skills and
influence to ensure that personnel and departments deliver the services their programs require. In this form of parallel organization,
the integrative managers rely upon *direct contact* with clinicians and
managers of other departments to gain their support and engage
their efforts. A typical use of direct contact is meeting with a physician to influence the physician's or the physician's associates' practice patterns, to encourage or plan for new areas of service, or to
obtain information about new technologies and services or their
financial implications. An integrative manager might also directly
contact a manager of a support service to resolve problems in scheduling, cost or quality of the service, or orientation of the staff in-
teracting with patients. With direct contact, the power of the
functional-department heads is not directly challenged. Direct contact, form 3, provides greater integration than forms 1 and 2. Compared to organizational forms further to the right along the
continuum, direct contact is limited in its ability to facilitate coordination of ongoing efforts because an integrative manager is the
only person who has any broad responsibility for each program.

In implementing the direct contact form of parallel organization and subsequent forms along the continuum of Figure 2.1,
two additional variations should be considered. First, a new department of integrative managers may or may not be established. Such

new integrative departments often result from transformation of staff functions such as marketing or planning, as described earlier. Establishing a new department makes a statement, lending credibility to the organization's increased emphasis on program integration. Alternatively, managers who have other responsibilities may assume additional integrative responsibilities, resulting in individuals' having dual jobs and responsibilities. Both the "new department" and "dual responsibility" variations provide a focus in an organization for each program and an individual who acts administratively on behalf of each program. Generally, medical staff find these arrangements to be a positive change, for they can more easily locate someone who can respond effectively to many of their concerns. Dual responsibilities are often confusing to members of the organization, however.

Neither variation necessarily evolves from a pure functional organization (form 1) through establishment of a new department (form 2) to assignment of integrative responsibilities with use of direct contact (form 3). Rather, a new department of integrative managers assigned to various programs can simply be established, or, alternatively, integrative responsibilities can simply be added to the roles of established management positions. Note also that head nurses and medical directors, particularly in specialized units, have some but not all of the integrative responsibilities and options of integrative managers. They are limited by position, by lack of legitimized responsibility for broad and farreaching integration, and often also by lack of management skills. In contrast, a vice president with dual responsibilities for hospital planning and for the administrative overview of a program, for example, typically carries the influence from his or her established position into the integrative program responsibilities. He or she generally is able to effect a response from support or clinical staff outside the unit more readily than a department head or nurse manager on a patient care unit could. However, when integrative managers are not directly involved in operations, they have limited opportunities to influence actual service delivery. The integrative manager's influence also is affected by the manager's skills and personality. (Selection of integrative managers, as well as ways to combine their responsibilities, will be discussed in greater detail in Chapter Three.)

Task Forces

Further along the continuum, at number 4 in Figure 2.1, the next variation of parallel organization involves formation of *task forces* of clinicians and managers from different functional departments and from the medical staff. The use of task forces, which by definition have a limited and relatively short life span (Charns and Schaefer, 1983, p. 156), allows input of multiple perspectives in decision making, thereby increasing the potential quality of those decisions. Through their interaction, members of a task force influence each other to support the program's purpose and objectives. Compared to direct contact, task forces are relatively more powerful for program integration and more threatening to the functional departments because a task force's influence on members of functional departments is, in fact, a loss of some control by the departments.

A typical application of a task force is planning a new service or program. For example, in planning activities for a trauma service, an integrative manager might involve key physicians and nurse managers from several specialties, as well as laboratory and radiology managers. If the planning leads to actual implementation, it also is valuable to include in the planning process those key people who will have responsibilities for implementation. Involving people in the planning contributes to their commitment to its successful implementation. (This point will be discussed in greater detail in Chapter Six.)

The integrative manager plays the key leadership role in a task force, initiating and facilitating meetings, representing the task force to the rest of the organization and its relevant publics, and managing conflicting perspectives of task force members. The integrative manager in this model also provides staff support to the task force, relying on his or her specialty skills (such as clinical expertise, marketing, or financial analysis). Thus, in addition to specialist skills, the integrative manager brings a generalist's orientation to the program and uses project management and conflict management as well as interpersonal skills. From extensive research of managers in similar positions in other industries, it is clear that the most effective integrators have strong interpersonal skills and their influence is based on their perceived competence (Lawrence and Lorsch, 1967, 1968; Charns, 1976).

Dedicated Personnel

The ease with which an integrative manager can influence other departments and gain their cooperation is enhanced when the other departments are reorganized into subunits that correspond to and are dedicated to the different programs (see form 5 in Figure 2.1). For example, specializing nursing units so that patients of any particular program are cared for on only one patient care unit (or, at most, on a few units) facilitates the coordinating efforts of the integrative manager by reducing the number of relationships to be managed and enhancing units' identification with programs and their goals. Dedicating social workers, dieticians, and other professionals to specified programs has a similar effect. Organizing and dedicating subunits within nonprofessional departments, such as housekeeping, to individual programs increases their integration into programs as well. This effect is enhanced further when each physician is involved with one or only a few programs and participates in program planning, evaluation, problem solving, and management decision making. When, in addition, patient care units are specialized by program, the benefits are compounded. By organizing this way, physicians and nurses can develop the type of effective working relationships that can occur only through frequent interaction. Such relationships are characterized by trust, flexibility, and valuing each other's contributions and perspectives. Note that these effects are built on collaboration and cooperation among people working toward shared goals, and do not depend on power, formal authority, or control.

Sometimes subdividing departments into units that correspond to different programs is not feasible, either because technological constraints or small size limit available organizing options. In such cases, it is helpful to have a department appoint individuals to serve as the primary contacts within their department for specific programs. Thus, for example, a cardiology liaison within the radiology department would represent the department to the cardiology program and would be its primary contact within radiology. The liaison person would learn the program's unique requirements, and would work to have the department meet the program's needs effectively, generally without referring requests to the top level of the department. Liaison people typically retain their regular responsibilities within their departments, and different people in a department serve as liaisons for different programs. The liaison people would also participate in their programs' problem-solving meetings, as necessary.

Teams

Form number 6 in Figure 2.1 is a stronger variation of the parallel organization. It calls for task forces to be developed into more permanent *teams,* having broader responsibilities and a longer tenure for the management of each program. The more permanent nature of teams makes them more powerful than task forces in influencing the behavior of their members. Therefore, teams are a greater threat to the control and influence of functional departments, as well as a more powerful mechanism for obtaining commitment to the programs. The comments regarding functioning of task forces and the skills and orientation of the integrative managers on task forces, described earlier, also apply to teams, but to an even greater extent. Teams represent a relatively greater degree of organizational commitment to programs, and because more time and effort are being applied to managing and coordinating programs, they are more costly to the organization. The payoff is the degree of focus, commitment, and coordination that is attained.

In the team approach, the integrative manager is usually either an administrator, with other limited responsibilities, or a clinician, such as a head nurse, who assumes program responsibilities in addition to functional responsibilities. The individual typically carries some personal influence from his or her functional line position. The balance of essential influence is derived through interpersonal skills and the credibility of the organization's program objectives. A head nurse typically helps coordinate care delivery with the best interests of patients and of the institution; expanding that role to one of following patients through the entire continuum of care and of influencing the delivery of services from the functional departments could favorably affect the effectiveness and efficiency of delivery of care. The integrative role need not be restricted only to nurse managers, however, and the advantages of using different types of integrative managers discussed under task forces apply equally well here.

Instead of one integrative manager, representatives from nursing management, the medical staff, and the administration can carry out this role. This trio may be led by one member of the group, or the authority may be divided among the three disciplines, depending on the nature of the issue at hand. Although such an arrangement is virtually never seen in other industries, the power distribution among medicine, nursing, and administration necessitates it in many health care organizations. This approach is more cumbersome than the single-manager structure, but it is often the only viable method of implementing a program team. The management group need not be restricted to people from nursing, medicine, and administration, nor need it be limited to trios. Other professions may be added or substituted, but the professions that are represented in the integrative management group should be those most centrally involved in the program. Increasing the size of the group allows for wider involvement within the organization, but increases the difficulty of managing the group itself.

Especially when using a trio, but also when using a single integrative manager having dual responsibilities of function and program, it is important to clearly delineate program responsibilities. This can be done by making the integrative manager accountable to a senior manager with broader, aggregate integrative responsibilities that cover several or all programs. Note that this is not a matrix. Rather, it is a parallel organization in which integrative managers are meeting two different types of responsibilities and are accountable to different people for them. The organization's commitment to the integrative responsibilities also should be shown by its evaluation and reward systems acknowledging integrative program management effectiveness.

The several forms of parallel organization represent, first, functions appended as new departments or roles and, then, increasing degrees of management focus, influence, coordination, and cost, as the programs overlie and affect the functional departments. The

relative strengths of a parallel organization, compared to other organizational alternatives, are that it retains clear lines of authority,
focuses management talent on market objectives, and encourages a
multidisciplinary approach. Among its weaknesses are that integrative managers do not control resources needed to deliver service, it
focuses program concerns without a direct mechanism for addressing them, it increases conflicting demands on functional departments, and it depends heavily on the skills and personal influence
of integrative managers.

In none of the forms of parallel organization structure is it
necessary to represent all potential programs with integrative managers or mechanisms. Typically, hospitals develop integrative managers, task forces, or teams for their most important programs,
where integration can greatly affect performance. Hospitals differ,
however, in what they consider important to performance. Some
have implemented integrating mechanisms to reach segments of
their market more effectively, and others have been focused on the
delivery of care. (We will discuss these differences in orientation in
detail in Chapter Seven.) Overall, then, integrating mechanisms
may directly affect only a portion of an organization's total activities. One hospital, for example, may have teams for oncology and
for cardiovascular services, a task force planning a new chronic back
pain program, a program manager using direct contact to coordinate ambulatory surgery, and no integrating mechanisms for other
services. The functions that are integrated in each program should
be determined based on program needs. Thus, all functions need
not be included. The strengths and limitations of the parallel structures will vary, then, with the degree to which they are implemented
in different parts of an organization.

In the middle of the continuum from functional to program organization is the matrix (number 7 in Figure 2.1). To gain an understanding of matrix organizations, however, it is best to jump to the far
end of the continuum and discuss program organizations first.

Program Organization

The program organization (number 9 in Figure 2.1) is made up of
program divisions, each of which includes all of the key personnel

required to deliver and manage its services. Emphasis is on relationships among specialists within each program. In theory, all of the functions directly involved in providing care for a given program would be contained within the program division. In other words, all key personnel would be accountable to their respective programs. (See Figure 2.3.)

In the pure program organization, each division is a "minihospital." The pure program organization could be implemented, for example, by a set of self-contained specialty hospitals, all operating under the name of a single hospital, with a single overall senior management team to which the individual hospitals reported, and with only support services, such as finance and personnel, provided by centralized staff groups. In practice, however, it is rarely feasible to duplicate all of the functional departments, as would be necessary to achieve the "pure" program organization form. This constraint is especially obvious when one considers duplicating expensive technologies. By assigning staff from a number of major professional and nonprofessional specialties to programs, and having these staff accountable not to a function but to their respective programs, the extreme form of program organization is approached. With this organization come most of the advantages and disadvantages noted earlier. Thus, in practice, many hospitals describing themselves as organized by programs actually have

Figure 2.3. Program Organization, Simplified Schematic.

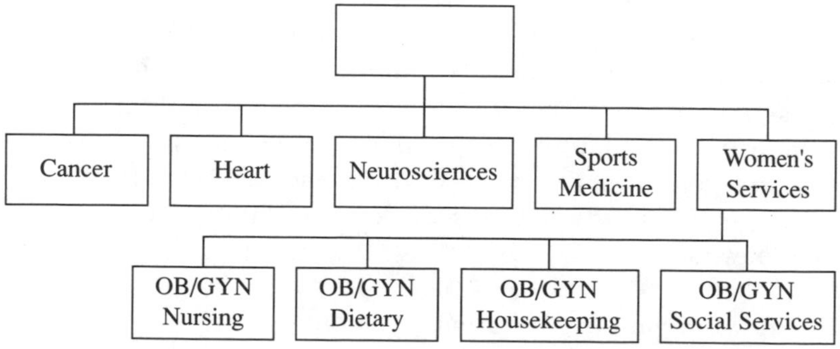

Note: Programs and functions shown are hypothetical.

many, but not all, staff, such as nurses, ultimately reporting to program managers rather than to their traditional professional function.

Program divisions may be strategic business units, but most likely are at least discrete cost centers. The strengths of a program organization include a management focus on individual programs' outputs, potential for role flexibility among disciplines, increased ease of measuring the costs of each program, the managerial ability to trade off cost and quality, the ability to plan the programs' business, focus on integrated service delivery, with potential for resource specialization by program, care process efficiencies, and responsiveness to the market or consumer. Weaknesses of the program organization include reduction in the ability to pool resources, resulting in loss of economies of scale by function, and reduction in control of organizationwide policies, with exceptions to standards advocated by programs. As shown in Figure 2.1, the program organization represents the ultimate trade-off of the traditional emphasis on individual functions and integration of functions within programs.

Two disadvantages of this organizational form should be noted. Just as the functional structure fosters territorialism by function and profession, the program organization fosters territorialism by program. Although this may not appear to be a great disadvantage, it can fragment care when a patient needs services of more than one program, and it encourages each program to focus on making its own decisions, independent of other programs. In addition, since nursing is typically the first department to be reorganized into programs, there is no longer a unified voice for the profession, and no strong organizational mechanism exists to take its place in maintaining professional competence. For these reasons and because the reorganization diminishes their power base, nursing leaders often strongly resist this kind of reorganization. When nursing is reorganized to report to another profession, the resulting subordination of nursing has dysfunctional consequences for both the hospital and the profession.

Modified Program Organization

Since no health care organization can afford to lose all of the advantages of a functional organization form, pure program structure is virtually never seen. The disadvantages of the program organization accrue for functions that are fragmented and self-contained within program divisions, even when not all functions are reorganized. Consequently, the pure program organization form provides an unacceptable balance between the form's advantages and disadvantages, and the pure form is not found in practice. Instead, most organizations that seek to maximize the advantages of the program organization form compensate for the form's disadvantages by having mechanisms for integrating the functions across program divisions. These represent a movement on the continuum of organizational configurations away from a pure program organization and toward a functional organization. This position is shown as number 8 on the continuum in Figure 2.1. For example, since in a pure program organization no departments would represent functions, no mechanism would exist to handle organizationwide professional nursing issues. To provide for this, a nurse executive might be appointed to oversee professional nursing issues, such as standards and in-service education, throughout the hospital. A nurse executive position could be augmented by a council consisting of nurses representing the different programs. Both of these mechanisms would be weaker and less influential than a department of nursing, since they lack direct control of operations, significant budget, or personnel issues. Similar arrangements might be developed for other functions and disciplines. The resulting modified program organization would provide some functional perspective, which the pure program organization does not. The modified program organization is found in practice, generally in large organizations that want to emphasize the program perspective over the functional perspective.

Matrix Organization

A true matrix organization (number 7 in Figure 2.1) provides balance between the strengths of the program and the functional forms. In a true matrix form, people and responsibilities are organized and managed in two dimensions simultaneously: a program organization is superimposed on a functional organization (see Figure 2.4). Davis and Lawrence (1979) note the following characteristics of a true matrix:

1. Approximately 15 to 20 percent of the members of the organization are responsible to more than one boss.
2. Influence is relatively balanced between the two dimensions (function and program).
3. Both bosses participate equally in subordinates' evaluations.

Figure 2.4. Matrix Organization, Simplified Schematic.

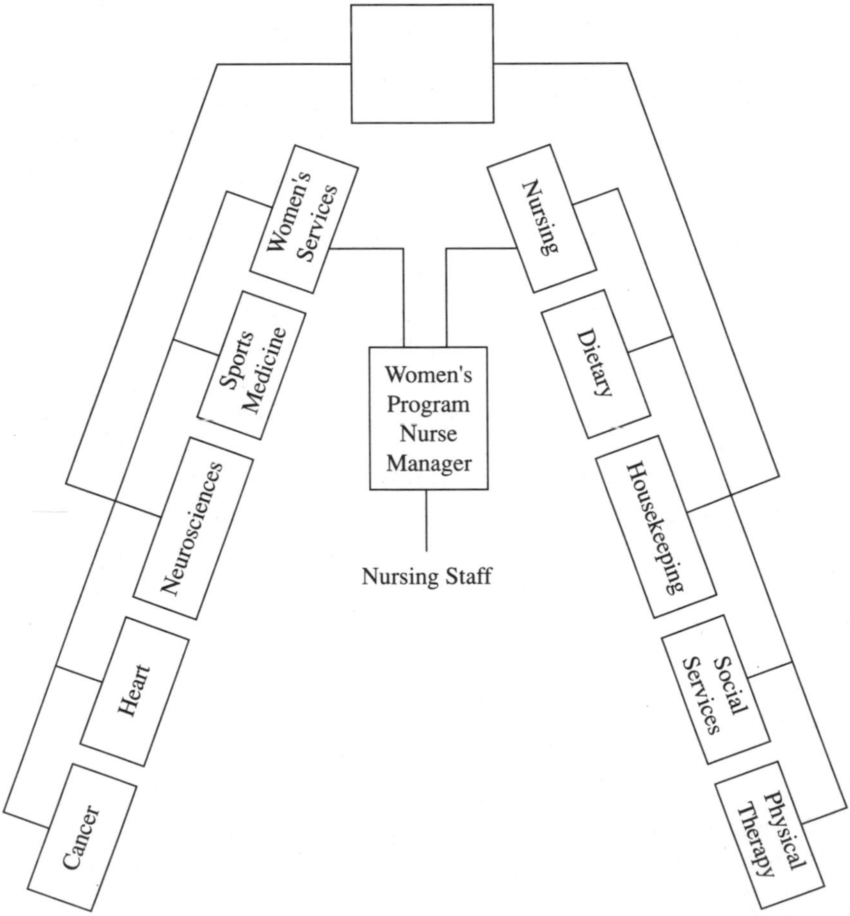

Note: Programs and functions represented are hypothetical.

4. Budgets are allocated by both function and program.
5. Both dimensions represent equally viable career paths.

The strengths of matrix organization are those of both the functional and the program forms; once consensus is achieved, there is strong commitment from the people involved; its flexibility allows shifts of emphasis as needs change. Its weaknesses are the increased potential for latent conflict to become manifest in the organization; the ambiguity inherent in dual reporting relationships; its increased managerial cost in time and personnel; and the difficulty of maintaining a true balanced matrix. It is unusual to find a hospital utilizing a matrix structure effectively. However, because the terminology is not used precisely in practice, many organizations with teams or task forces refer to themselves incorrectly, as matrix organizations.

Conclusion

This chapter has presented the continuum of organizational forms, described the prototypical structures along the continuum, and discussed each structure's inherent strengths and weaknesses. In the following chapters, additional aspects of making the various forms operational and selecting the appropriate form to address a hospital's particular needs will be presented. In addition, characteristics of effective integrative managers and the uses of reward, evaluation, control, and information systems to support the various forms of integrative management will be discussed. The case studies in subsequent chapters will provide detailed applications of these concepts and additional guidance in choosing the appropriate organizational arrangements.

Chapter Three

Leadership Skills
for Integrative
Managers

The success of many efforts has been deemed to be "a function of the people involved." The "best laid plans" and superior strategies notwithstanding, there remains a dependency on the quality of the individuals responsible for steering the effort. The purpose of this chapter is to discuss the type of individuals who work best in integrative management positions. It is not true that all you need is good people; you need good people with specific skills, abilities, and orientations, who can be effective integrators, and these people need appropriate systems and organizational support.

Matching the Strategy and Structure with the Integrator

As discussed in Chapter Two, structure should match strategy; in other words, form should follow function. (This relationship will be discussed further in Chapter Seven.) In presenting the alternative organization designs, we noted unavoidable, inherent ambiguity in authority and power in several of the structures. Managing effectively within those structures requires a high tolerance for ambiguity, as well as excellent skills at conflict management and interpersonal communication. These requirements are not as great in the pure functional and augmented functional structures, nor in the pure program organization, however. Therefore, it also is critically important to match the individual—in terms of skills, experience, and personality—with the organization structure in which he or she must work. Thus, prior to determining who will fill various integrative management positions, it is critical to decide the form of the organization in terms of the continuum presented in Figure 2.1. Will the use of task forces be sufficient to attain the desired outcomes? Or will the establishment of permanent teams provide the required consistency? Is the organization sophisticated enough and does it need a matrix structure to ensure adequate emphasis on both function and program? Or is the organization large enough—and can it afford to lose advantages of the functional focus—to utilize a program organization?

In an organization as complex as a hospital, people rarely have complete control over all of the things they are responsible to manage. Most notably, since physicians determine the course of treatment, and thus directly affect resource utilization, managers do not have direct control over major clinical expenses. Managers, however, can influence clinicians directly, as well as affect the organizational context in which they practice, by promoting the value and importance of cost consciousness as well as the coordination and efficiency of care delivery. The integrative managers' ability to do these things effectively depends on their influence, which is affected by both organizational and personal factors. An organization can provide a basis for influence by granting a person formal authority. Where managers do have formal authority, as in program divisions operating as strategic business units, they can control many expenses, and may directly affect revenue through changes in services and prices. In contrast, integrative managers in parallel structures are given little or no formal control over expenses and no formal authority over personnel. In organizations where integrative managers are held accountable for profit, it is especially important that they hold sufficient power to influence decisions on both revenues and expenses. Since by design the structure does not provide this basis of influence, other factors are extremely important.

The education and experience required of individuals depends on the organizational form. Program organizations (numbers 8 and 9 on the continuum) and matrix organizations (number 7) require individuals trained and experienced as senior level managers, with broad organizational perspectives and, typically, also with strong clinical backgrounds. Inherent in the position of program manager in these organizations is a fairly high degree of formal authority. Compared to other organizational forms, the matrix and program divisional forms provide program managers more formal power; thus those managers rely less on informal influence.

In the task force and team approaches, managers must be able to utilize various kinds of formal and informal influence. These abilities are often difficult to outline in the skill requirement section of a job description and are certainly difficult to overtly plan as part of a strategy. In this chapter, we will delineate the characteristics individuals need in order to serve as effective managers in the various organization structures, advocating for their programs and integrating the variety of functions and disciplines on which the programs depend.

Skills That Integrators Need

Effective integrators need a blend of skills drawn from two categories: content and process skills. Content skills apply in the more technical areas, such as planning, finance, marketing, and operations, as well as in particular clinical areas or specialties, such as orthopedics or cardiovascular disease. In contrast, the process skills can be seen as the "soft" skills that include active listening, managing effective group process, influencing, understanding and utilizing the change process, and being able to encourage participation, cooperation, and visioning. Effective integrators have strong listening skills and are able to understand viewpoints very different from their own and to reconcile diverse opinions. Because their orientations are balanced, they can exemplify their interest in representing the issues broadly, as opposed to acting out of self-interest or with a biased perspective. An integrator's credibility depends on others' perceiving him or her as exemplifying an understanding and valuing of other individuals' issues. By using effective process skills—

consulting with or involving other individuals on issues that are important to them—an integrator builds confidence and trust.

Where the requirement for integration of disciplines is limited, content or technical skills are often a major factor in determining the choice of integrative managers. In a purely functional structure, no integrator roles exist. In parallel structures, from direct contact (number 3 in Figure 2.1) through team approaches (number 6), integrative managers need both intense content and process skills. Integrators must earn their influence and credibility by being seen as effective leaders and being looked to for content and process guidance. In program organizations (numbers 8 and 9), program managers are likely to be surrounded by other managers who have strong content skills, and therefore the process skills are typically more critical for success.

Content Skills

Content skills are needed both for making specific content-related decisions and as an important basis for earning credibility from peers and associates. An effective way to gain credibility quickly in the health care industry is to have the clinical expertise required to understand and resolve patient care issues. For this reason, nursing managers often are able to serve as effective integrators. To the integrative role they bring prior relationships with physicians and other clinical managers, skills in problem identification and resolution, and a holistic perspective on patient care needs. Even though many barriers separate the different disciplines in health care, an integrator can reach common ground by bringing the focus on any issue back to the patients and what is best for them. The use of this focus when determining the best options during problem resolution contributes greatly to reducing tensions and increasing cooperation. In some problem-solving efforts, the "customer" may not be a patient, but rather a physician, an outside agency, or a department within the organization. Placing the emphasis on the customer's needs can focus a group with diverse perspectives.

Through management education and experience, a clinically trained manager can learn to effectively use the key disciplines of planning, marketing, and finance. One approach that complements the clinical manager is to have the planning, marketing, and finance experts work together as a team with the clinical manager to identify opportunities, strategies, problems, and solutions. The planning, marketing, and finance experts focus their energies on the program and services at hand, while the clinical manager interprets the "business" disciplines and assimilates them into the management of the effort. The clinical manager also often serves as the bridge and translator between the people in the business disciplines and the clinically trained individuals in the organization.

Thus, individuals' clinical skills gain them immediate credibility with the other professionals in the planning or problem-solving effort. This includes physicians, who are key players in the development of innovation in health care organizations. However, the business skills—planning, finance, and marketing—are critical and also must be represented. An integrative manager may have a solid understanding of a specific clinical area and of the many technical skills needed. If not, however, dedicated support from the business professionals can complement the efforts of clinically oriented managers. For example, one hospital, very successful in its implementation of programs, assigned a member of the finance staff to each program. Each finance expert focused on the one program, participated with the clinically trained program management team, and developed an effective relationship that bridged historical misunderstandings and past tensions. Over time and with a planned management development program, clinical managers usually will grasp the business disciplines. However, it may not be necessary for each integrative manager to be an expert in all disciplines as long as the needed expertise is available.

Collaboration Between Technical Experts and Integrators

Collaboration between integrators and planning, marketing, and finance experts that brings integrators exposure to new skills and perspectives works best if it is a deliberate and well-understood effort. All the people involved need to be willing to share information and learn from one other. The collaboration should not be interpreted by any technical expert as an opportunity to gain access to (or power over) the clinical contingency. Rather, technical experts should see it as a way to share technical logic and advice with individuals who have the credibility and influence to get clinicians to listen and to assess and form actions to resolve or respond to a financial, marketing, or planning problem or opportunity.

We have seen technical experts use the relationship in both ways, leading to vastly different outcomes. The technical expert who values the relationship with integrators and recognizes his or her own limitations, in terms of communicating with the clinical world, earns trust, cooperation, and respect from integrators and their constituents. This technical expert sees the relationship as interdependent and promotes the development of a productive and effective liaison. Obviously, to achieve this cooperative stance, integrators must view the relationship in the same light. Although the effort is energy intensive and time consuming, the quality and quantity of the outcomes are excellent.

An example of effectively managing the relationship is a financial analyst who spent hours working with a clinical integrative manager to help the manager understand how information was gathered, what it represented, and what conclusions could be assessed from the information. The integrative manager was then able to use the information in explaining to a group of clinical professionals that the length of stay for patients with certain specific diagnoses had been creeping up. As a result, the physicians decided to analyze utilization data to understand the causes of the increasing lengths of stay. The problem was well received, and the physicians were engaged in understanding the causes, knowing that their practice patterns could be contributing to the problem. Thus, the issue that concerned the financial analyst was communicated to clinicians in a nonthreatening way by a trusted individual (the integrator), and action was taken by those most directly capable of modifying practice to resolve the problem.

A technical expert who does not value relationships with integrators as partnerships and who uses integrators to gain a platform with the clinical constituency will most undoubtedly encounter resistance, skepticism, and lack of commitment for proposed resolutions. Trust levels wane rather than grow, leading to compromised quantity and quality of outcomes. When participants develop "ground rules" for making decisions, a structured process can be established that may alleviate their frustration. In the former example, with the expert and integrator who respect the partnership, ground rules grew and developed naturally. In the case of a technical expert and an integrator who do not mutually value the partnership, time and energy must be committed to purposeful negotiation and identification of roles and responsibilities.

A common example of an ineffective partnership can be found in the experience of a marketing expert who made decisions about what particular service to promote and how to promote it. She did not consult with the integrator or with the other clinical professionals involved with the program when she planned a promotion campaign. When she presented her concept to the integrator, she met resistance instead of support, and a power struggle began. The marketing expert had lost ground in terms of credibility and trust with the integrator. The concept to be marketed, even though a sound one, was put in jeopardy as a result of the integrator's feelings of lack of control. It was necessary for the marketing expert to backtrack several steps in the concept development in order to engage the interest and support of the integrator and other clinicians. The final concept was slightly modified, but the stress and strain on relationships and the involved individuals' reduced productivity was evident.

We have observed that technical experts who recognize the value of a collaborative relationship with integrators and clinicians are secure in their own position and believe in "earned influence." In contrast, technical experts who do not value partnership relationships typically are fighting for or expect to utilize direct power that is attributed to their position within the organization and do not perceive the importance of earning influence and credibility.

Process Skills

The more difficult set of skills to develop are the process skills. Relatively intangible and often not the focus of formal education, their importance is sometimes difficult for individuals to appreciate. This is especially true for individuals who have had little prior exposure to process issues and process skill development. Such is the case with traditional medical education. However, the effective development and use of process skills are crucial factors in gaining informal credibility in an organization. The ability to get things done through and with other people, and to gain cooperation and commitment to a project or the resolution of a problem, is an almost sure route to gaining credibility and thus influence. Some individuals feel they need formal authority to get their job done. Other managers recognize the blessings and importance of informal influence and are able to function very well in a position with little or no formal authority.

In other industries, "traditional" product managers have no formal authority but a lot of responsibility for making their products profitable by meeting the needs of their customers, producing efficiently, and marketing and selling in the right markets. They play an integrative role that is seen to be effective training for executive positions. An important reason, we believe, that many executives come from integrative positions is that they develop and use process skills in those jobs that guarantee their credibility and their ability to engage the cooperation of various experts in the organization. This can be paralleled in health care; integrative management positions can be used as a training ground for developing senior managers.

Use of Existing Managers as Integrators

It often is difficult to find effective integrative managers. In addition, when a position is new and must be introduced, its function and realm of influence are likely to be unclear to other people in the organization. Furthermore, many organizations cannot justify the salary expense for full-time integrators in addition to their existing management group. One approach that has been successful in addressing these issues is to give managers who have strong track records for effective teamwork and leadership additional responsibilities as integrators. These managers bring not only their personal influence to the integrative position but also the influence and direct authority of the other position for which they are still responsible. In the evolution of their relationships within the organization, effective managers develop and utilize competence-based influence. Established managers who are recognized and respected in an organization as a result of their effective use of a combination of clinical (content) skills and process skills have a head start in building credibility. They are likely to already have the relationships with many physicians and managers that would give them informal influence. Each success demonstrates the value and competence of the integrator and the process, from which additional influence for both grows. For example, the nursing director for an orthopedic unit typically has the physician relations, technical competence, and organizational recognition to be an effective integrator for the orthopedic service. In addition, he or she has the clinical "name tag" that assures medically and clinically oriented colleagues that the focus on patient care will not be jeopardized.

Organizations have used existing managers as integrators in two ways. One way is to recruit them into new integrative positions and relieve them of their previous responsibilities. Although this is more straightforward and "cleaner" than having dual roles and responsibilities, the integrative position may not initially demand a full-time commitment. Thus, some institutions have achieved success by giving individuals an integrative role as a second role, in addition to the person's other responsibilities. Often the integrative responsibilities require relating to many of the same people and overlap with the integrator's other position.

There are some problems with giving responsibility for two roles to one individual, however. The individual may tend to fall back on the first role in times of stress and when the work load is heavy, or the individual may not be able to spend the time that is needed on the original responsibilities. Ambiguity in roles may develop, and the individual who has low tolerance for ambiguity may feel immobilized. Other individuals may show uncooperative tendencies owing to feelings of envy or insecurity. New communication links tend to form that modify the integrator's patterns of interaction and relationships, leaving people previously in frequent contact with the manager with the feeling that they are being left out. Uncooperative or negative reactions may result.

However, combining roles can be an extremely effective way of building innovative organizational arrangements. Recognizing the downside of this approach and creatively dealing with some of the fallout through specialized types of support can help to achieve success. For example, a nursing director who takes on an integrative role may need the support of a resource person, who would take on some of the routine operational duties. Developing the skills of an assistant to plan staffing, conduct quality assurance audits, and follow up on minor problems can be an effective way to groom new managers and allow integrators more time away from their routine operational duties.

Involvement of Senior Managers

Individuals designing an integrative structure for an institution must decide how high in the organization to go to gain the attention and credibility required for the change effort. One way of getting the necessary attention is to involve members of senior management. The senior managers have substantial direct power and influence to get things done, and their involvement signals to the rest of the institution the importance of the effort. In moving toward integrative configurations on the organizational continuum, it becomes increasingly critical to heighten the involvement of senior managers.

In program organizational forms (numbers 8 and 9 in Figure 2.1), the integrative manager is *by design* a senior manager responsible for an entire program division. An organization can only achieve a true matrix (number 7) by balancing influence between the departments and programs. Therefore, a manager of at least departmental status is needed in the program management positions in a matrix. In task force (number 4) through team approaches (number 6), senior managers can either serve as integrative managers themselves or can provide support and advice through membership on the program task forces or teams. Unless senior managers act in unsupportive ways as members of an integrative group, both methods indicate the importance of the effort to the organization. Having senior managers serve as integrative managers in the direct contact alternative (number 3) also lends greater influence to that integrative position.

Because direct contact is more limited in its integrative potential than task forces and other structures further to the right on the organizational continuum, an organization selecting direct contact should question whether it truly wants to staff the integrative positions with senior managers. It is important to do so when direct contact is planned as the first step in implementing integrative structures, with more powerful structural alternatives to be implemented in the future. Especially in the early stages of evolution to a parallel structure, it is effective to involve senior managers and have them interface directly with physicians. This signals the importance of the effort and demonstrates their commitment to the new approach. Senior managers' early involvement and communication also help to reduce resistance and gain the commitment of other hospital managers.

Senior managers with operational positions who are given integrative roles will face the same problems differentiating between roles as do more junior managers. Subordinates of senior managers may also feel a lack of attention and support. This may be heightened by changes in responsibilities; although they actually are critical to the organization's effectiveness, they no longer appear central to it. It is important to recognize staff and support them through these adjustments so that both the traditional operational and the innovative integrative responsibilities are achieved.

In much of this chapter, we have implicitly focused on organizations that are somewhere on the continuum between direct contact (number 3) and teams (number 6). Occasionally, however, a radical restructuring into a program organization (number 8 or 9) is called for. Such major change risks tremendous resistance and turnover within the clinical components of the organization. Since nursing is more affected by radical restructuring, and a strong advocate for nursing and other professional issues is needed, the organization should consider seeking a nurse to be chief operating officer. The nurse executive should have a broad background that includes the development of the business skills that can be achieved through an integrative position, as described above. The exposure, experience, and organizational philosophy gained by integrators can serve to mold a different type of chief operating officer who can maintain a balance within the organization.

Triad Management

Another method of achieving integrative program management is the establishment of triads, or trios. These are program management groups composed of a physician, a nurse, and an administrator. The three triad members each retain their traditional management and clinical responsibilities and are also jointly accountable for their program. Thus, for example, the nurse manager in a triad for a cardiovascular services program continues to be responsible for nursing personnel and quality of nursing care on units caring for cardiology patients, but also shares responsibility with a physician leader and an administrator for the performance of the cardiovascular program.

Triads provide an effective vehicle for collaborative decision making among the leadership of the three major constituencies in each program. Whereas in traditionally structured organizations nursing, medicine, and administration each independently make substantial management decisions that affect programs, the triad structure encourages joint decision making and consideration of the relationships among all aspects of each program. For example, in traditional hospital structures, budget requests are submitted separately for medicine, nursing, and administrative components. In triads, these requests can be coordinated, and a consolidated budget request for the program can be proposed.

Because it adds the complications inherent in group dynamics, the triad approach can be cumbersome. It also carries the potential for staff assigned to a program, as well as other managers, to play one triad member off against another. However, if effective collaboration among the disciplines is attained, triads can vastly improve understanding between disciplines, provide a perspective that encompasses the total management of the program, and achieve integrated, balanced decisions. When triads attain a high level of effectiveness, this contributes to acceptance of the approach by the whole organization.

Where this has worked well, physician-manager positions are paid rather than voluntary. Paying physicians provides a reasonable incentive to commit time and indicates that the organization values the physician-management position. Team-building exercises also are effective for developing credible relations and respect among the three individuals, who come from diverse backgrounds and training experiences. Although power is said to be equal among the team members, in effective triads members clearly and freely defer to different professionals, depending on the subject at hand.

A critical element in the triad approach is recognition of and commitment to the triads as vehicles for integrating and decision making. Where the triad approach has been tried and has not worked well, senior management has not been committed to it. Thus, all of the major constituencies involved were not committed to the triads' success. Individuals within triads tended to give lip service to the integrative effort and to continue to do "business as usual." To avoid this, incentives and expectations for the triads must be established and communicated. For example, in one institution, the executive management group frowned on the triads' bringing them stalemated issues for resolution. Each triad was held accountable as a group, and soon learned that they were seen as ineffective if they could not resolve issues at their own levels. Thus, they began to work harder to reach consensus. Additionally, triad members must communicate among themselves and develop a level of trust that precludes others from taking advantage by means of evasive action, or "end-runs." Triads must be seen to be and must operate as true teams in order to get the proper respect and credibility from other components of the organization.

Community hospitals that typically have unpaid physician chiefs may find the triad approach prohibitive from an expense standpoint. Alternatively, they can use a team approach for coordinating the necessary disciplines, which most likely will go far beyond medicine, nursing, and administration. They then can utilize the physicians in a consultative manner through individual or group meetings. Team approaches such as this one may only require two to five hours per month from the representative physician(s). Although not as strong an integrative management vehicle as a triad, a multidisciplinary team that includes physician involvement is a positive approach to achieving needed coordination and commitment.

Conclusion

The major points raised and discussed in this chapter can be summarized as follows:

1. Structure must follow strategy. Consider what is to be achieved and then design a structure that supports achievement of those goals.

2. The structure chosen to meet the particular strategy should dictate many of the qualifications needed for integrative management positions.

3. Effective integrators need a mix of skills that fall into two general categories: content (or technical) skills and process skills. Influence and credibility are earned by integrative managers according to the skills they possess and the use they make of them.

4. Clinically trained managers often make effective integrators because of their credibility and existing relationships with other clinicians. Technical skills, such as finance and marketing, can be obtained through effective partnerships formed with individuals who have those skills.

5. Integrative managers and technical managers must value collaboration and establish mutual respect and trust.

6. Established managers can be given additional responsibilities as integrators. Methods of supporting these individuals must be designed to allow time and provide rewards for the integrative activities. Downfalls of this approach include the potential for integrators to concentrate on their traditional roles.

7. Senior managers are required as integrators in some approaches. In others, their support and involvement are needed to communicate to the institution the importance of the effort and to empower the integrative managers.

8. Strong process and interpersonal skills are essential for integrative managers, especially in structures where their formal authority is limited. Credibility can be earned and cooperation gained through strong process skills.

Chapter Four

Reward Systems
That Support
Integrative Management
and Change

"Organizations would be simple to run if it weren't for the people." More than one manager has said something akin to this when faced with organizational problems such as lack of responsiveness to patients, quality problems, or low productivity, or when trying to implement an organizational change. The facts are that organizations are made up of people, and the behavior of an organization is the aggregate of the behaviors of the people who work in it. People in integrative organizations must behave differently than people in traditional organizations do. In our experience in implementing integrative management, most of the time and effort required for the change is devoted to redirecting the behavior of the people in the organization. Understanding how rewards affect people is a key factor in implementing and maintaining effective integrative structures.

By influencing rewards through both direct and indirect means, managers can have substantial impacts on how people behave. Often, managers unintentionally encourage behavior that works against the best interests of their organization. They also often overlook the potential use of organizational rewards to encourage desired behavior. The effective implementation of integrative arrangements in health care organizations depends on the behavior of a number of key people. Thus, an organization that encourages behavior that does not support the integrative structure will, at best, not be able to reap the full potential of these new organization and management practices and, at worst, will create an ambiguous situation that is dysfunctional, both for the people in the organization and for achieving the organization's desired outcomes.

The general subject of motivation and rewards has been the focus of numerous books and articles. In fact, it is one of the central topics in any basic course on organizational behavior. In this chapter we will briefly describe the relationships between rewards and behavior, and will concentrate on the application of reward systems to support implementation of integrative arrangements.

Motivation and Rewards

In our experience in all kinds of organizations, including health care, we have observed that there are two kinds of people: those who obviously are highly goal driven and achievement oriented and those who aren't. We have had success as well as trouble with both. The goal-oriented people typically are highly motivated and exhibit high energy. Sometimes, however, that energy is not directed where the organization needs to go. Their high energy level and commitment to goals other than the organization's (or the organizational change program) can be substantial barriers to innovation.

For example, consider the case of a hospital department head, Mark Mann, who has spent many years developing what he considers to be a top-notch professional department. It is recognized by the profession, and the professional community regards it as an excellent place to work. Mark takes pride in the department and in his accomplishment building it. Over the years the hospital has formally acknowledged and rewarded Mark for the professional environment he has built and for achieving goals he set for recruitment and retention. Recently, Jerry Jones, chief operating officer (COO), suggested changing the organization so that staff from the various professional departments would be dedicated to different programs (number 5 on the organizational continuum Figure 2.1). The integrative program managers report directly to Jerry. Both Jerry and Mark report to the chief executive officer (CEO). Mark has resisted the change. He believes it will remove his control and splinter his department, and no amount of persuasion can seem to convince him otherwise. In fact, speaking privately to Mark, other department heads have called the organizational change unfair and said they support his position.

These perceptions and the behaviors that are related to them should not come as a surprise to the CEO, COO, or reader. Mark is not acting irrationally or being unnecessarily stubborn. In any situation, complex forces act on the people involved and influence their behavior. Many previous actions and events reinforce a particular way of looking at things and doing things, leading an individual to believe that is how he or she should behave. In Mark's situation, there are few forces, inducements, rewards, or new goals to redirect his energies and attention. Therefore, why should he change his behavior and support the new approach? Often, a request from the COO or CEO is simply not enough. In fact, in this situation, Jerry, the COO and Mark's organizational peer, may be seen as a competitor for power, whose requests Mark will deny (typically in a masked, organizationally acceptable way).

Not only has a history of reinforcement encouraged Mark to act in a particular way but also few if any of the other rewards have changed. First, the CEO has not asked directly for new behaviors. By enlisting Mark's support for the implementation of the new organizational goals and vision, the CEO could provide Mark with a new, legitimate, and rewarding focus for his energies and talents. However, even if the CEO makes such an effort, Mark still may not "get the message." One important reason is that many significant events in organizations—such as personnel evaluations, goal setting, planning, and budgeting—occur in annual cycles. People typically have to go through at least one, if not several, confirming events, such as evaluations, before they believe the new way of doing things is real. When these events do occur in annual cycles, the time required to implement new behaviors is extended. Of course, it is also possible to change processes, such as review of goals and evaluation, to a higher frequency. Then, confirmation of the expected new behaviors could be given in perhaps three months, rather than a year.

In many situations we have seen a CEO, who is a legitimate authority figure, withhold public support for the new organizational design. This leaves others in the organization not knowing which way the "political winds" are blowing and how important it really is to support the new arrangements. Sometimes the cause of a CEO's hesitancy reflects a desire not to "play parent" by resolving the "squabble among siblings" (immediate subordinates). Sometimes it stems from a desire to avoid confronting a department head. The fact is, however, that the more highly motivated the department heads are, the harder they will work to protect the status quo, which is what the current rewards encourage, and the more they will appear stubborn and resistant to change—unless their motivation is redirected toward supporting the new organization.

Another important aspect of Mark's situation is that the indicators of organizational power have not changed. Typically, managers measure the amount of their power by the size of their budgets and the number of people in their control. Not wanting to lose power, why should Mark want to diminish control over some of his people? Peer pressure from the other department heads to not break ranks and give in to a change that is seen to adversely affect all of them also affects Mark's behavior. In this sense, Mark is avoiding a sanction (a negative reward) by resisting the change. Eliminating the organization's formal reinforcement of the old goals and behaviors is insufficient to bring about the desired change, because many other forces work to maintain the status quo. A new shared vision and set of goals are needed to redirect the efforts of Mark and his peers.

In contrast to managers like Mark are individuals who are not goal driven and do not appear very motivated. As a result, they rarely attain positions of authority. However, they may have a significant influence on the services the organization provides and its contact with the public. One example of this type of person is a dietary service worker in a large hospital we visited recently, as part of a site review for a major grant. All through the day the senior managers made themselves available to the site visit team, told us they would help us with anything we wanted, and cleared their schedules to ensure their ability to respond to our needs. In the afternoon, the site visit team asked if we might remain in a small dining room after our late lunch for a private discussion. A few minutes after the senior executives left the room, a dietary worker came in to clear the tables. We asked for just a few minutes alone and were told, "Oh, no. I'm sorry I can't do that. I get off at two o'clock." All of the senior managers' efforts toward hospitality were diminished in ten seconds by this remark.

Some might say this person was not motivated. On the contrary, she was very motivated, but her motivation was to leave by two o'clock. Unfortunately, her motivation was not directed in a way that would further the organization's goals.

It is highly unusual for a person not to be motivated at all. Something motivates nearly every one of us. Perhaps it is achievement, power, peer pressure, recognition, or the joy of doing a particular activity. What is at issue is whether the factors that motivate a person encourage organizationally desirable behavior, undesirable behavior, or behavior that has nothing to do with the organization.

Intrinsic Rewards

Generally speaking, there are two types of rewards: intrinsic and extrinsic. Simply stated, intrinsic rewards are inherent in a particular activity. For example, many people find playing video games or listening to music intrinsically rewarding. Work itself often is intrinsically rewarding and is what has attracted many people to a particular field or profession. Intrinsic rewards can be extremely powerful motivators because the rewards are direct. No outside intervention is needed for an individual to get intrinsic rewards from an activity. The power of intrinsic rewards is demonstrated by the tenacity with which some people play video games or push themselves to complete crossword puzzles and other games.

In organizations there are two major considerations with regard to intrinsic rewards. The first is whether the activity furthers organizational goals. The second is how the organization facilitates or hinders people in accomplishing their work.

An employee playing video games at work may be receiving intrinsic rewards, but the organization is not gaining from those efforts. Similarly, an organization does not gain from an employee's performing an activity that no longer is needed but which the employee finds enjoyable. The key in these examples is for the organization to motivate people to perform needed work by making it intrinsically rewarding. To do so, Hackman and Oldham (1975) suggest redesigning jobs to increase five core dimensions: skill variety, task identity, task significance, autonomy, and feedback.

A related example is characterized by displaced goals. Here, the goals of an individual or part of the organization take on greater importance than the goals of the total organization. A well-known example in the organizational literature is the librarian who does not want to lend out books because doing so means they will not be available for other borrowers. This is obviously irrational from the perspective of the overall goals of the library, but is quite rational when seen from the narrower perspective of optimizing availability. Another example is a job placement counselor who does not share job opportunities with other counselors in the office so that she can keep them for her clients. This practice allows the one counselor to make more job placements and to gain satisfaction from her work by doing so. However, the restriction of information negatively affects the placement agency's ability to place as many clients in appropriate jobs as is possible (Blau, 1955).

The second consideration is whether an organization interferes with an individual performing a worthwhile activity, thereby reducing its inherent reward. For example, nursing staff often are frustrated that other departments are not more responsive to their needs and patients' needs, or that short staffing requires them to reduce time with their patients. As a result, they find the intrinsic rewards in their work are reduced, and burnout may occur. Included in this category are any individuals whose ability to do their jobs well depends on others. The critical issue is how the organization can facilitate rather than hinder accomplishment of work that furthers organizational goals.

Integrative management does provide mechanisms to do exactly this. Since the programs provide a basis for coordination of services, increase general awareness of the need for responsiveness to patients, and provide a vehicle for obtaining resources, the integrative arrangements have the potential for increasing intrinsic rewards. Many staff who have worked in integrative organizations report greater satisfaction because they are better able to be responsive to the needs of their patients.

When an organization is implementing an integrative structure, however, its benefits initially may not be apparent to many staff. Therefore, they may not perceive the new arrangements as rewarding and, in turn, may resist them. Although integrative management is usually implemented for "good" reasons, most people in an organization do not know that or do not see the reasons in the same way. Therefore, a critical step in implementing integrative arrangements is to establish the need for the change so that people will give the new arrangements a try. We will return to the subject of implementation of change in Chapter Six.

Extrinsic Rewards

Extrinsic rewards are provided to a person for behaving in a particular way or for achieving an outcome. Many but not all of an individual's extrinsic rewards are controlled by an organization. Most people are quite attentive to extrinsic rewards, and they can be a powerful influence on behavior. A key to the effective use of extrinsic rewards is to link rewards directly to desired behaviors or outcomes. If people do not know that a reward is contingent upon a particular behavior or outcome, they will not be motivated by that reward to behave in the desired way.

Thus, a critical management activity is conveying to subordinates what behaviors and outcomes are desired and backing these up with organizational rewards that are highly valued by the individuals. By establishing explicit goals and relating them to rewards, an individual's motivation can be directed at organizationally desirable activities. This is a powerful motivator. When the outcomes that are the basis of rewards are measurable, and concrete information is provided on an individual's performance, the impact on behavior is further reinforced. As one CEO noted the first year after a financial bonus was instituted, "I will never forget how Tony's [the COO] eyes lit up when I handed him his bonus check." The economic value of the bonus is certainly important, but so is the symbolic value conveyed by the reward. It reinforces the goals, says the organization is really serious about them, and acknowledges their accomplishment.

An important factor to consider in regard to extrinsic rewards is that people can only focus on a limited number of desired outcomes and behaviors. Those that are emphasized by the organization will generally get people's attention to the exclusion of others. Applied too strictly, the use of extrinsic rewards can encourage dysfunctional behavior. For example, if the manager of Central Sterile Supply is measured and rewarded only on keeping inventory costs low, he or she most likely will control supplies so tightly that they may actually be unavailable when they are needed. When performance assessment is based on only a few indicators, they will get the employee's attention to the exclusion of other, possibly more important, issues.

Confusion over job priorities can also occur when managers reward one behavior while hoping for another (Kerr, 1975). For example, in universities it is relatively easy to count the number of publications produced by faculty members, but it is difficult to get reliable assessments of teaching effectiveness. Thus, even when a university wishes to encourage teaching excellence, it often falls into the trap of rewarding research publication to the exclusion of teaching. This is reinforced by a history of tenure being granted for research, with rare exceptions of faculty being promoted for outstanding teaching. Some universities actually monitor the number of pages of faculty publications. This, of course, encourages verbosity rather than concise writing.

One closed-panel health maintenance organization (HMO), in which medical staff were paid a salary, was concerned with physician productivity. The HMO instituted a system to determine a portion of compensation based upon each physician's efforts, as measured by patient office visits. The initial reaction of the medical staff was anger toward HMO administration. Many then noted that they could easily affect the number of office visits without increasing the number of patients in their panel (practice). They would simply see more simple cases, such as colds. This would increase patient visits, although not the number of people being cared for, but it would also increase laboratory and other diagnostic procedures, supply utilization, and work load of other staff. The new reward system was destined to increase costs rather than increase true productivity.

Rewards that everybody gets—system rewards—are not as powerful motivators as rewards that are contingent on an individual's performance. System rewards encourage people to join an organization and remain in its employ. For example, consider the state hospital discussed in Chapter One, where excellent salaries and benefits encouraged staff to remain employed there, even though it was professionally unrewarding. System rewards, however, do not directly encourage hard work or efforts directed at organizational goals. Rewards that are directly related to accomplishments and behavior have a greater impact on quantity and quality of work.

In a large hospital that prided itself on caring for its staff and that did not terminate employees for inadequate performance, we found many people whose behavior was inhibiting the hospital's effectiveness. Several were in the Admitting Department, where staff kept track of bed availability with little pieces of paper. Finding beds for urgent admissions was difficult and inefficient, which led to patients' being placed temporarily, only to be transferred fairly soon to a more appropriate unit than the one they were initially admitted to. Only a handful of staff really knew how the system worked, and over the years they had done many favors for some "favorite" physicians when those doctors needed patients admitted. Changing the admitting process presented a major challenge to the hospital's senior management. Examination of the reward system provides some insights into why it was so hard to change.

The organization did not reward members of the Admitting Department for efficiency or overall responsiveness to patients. Nor did it provide negative feedback on poor performance. Salary increases and continued employment were not contingent on work performance, and everyone in the hospital knew this. The fact that formal evaluation and rewards were unrelated to work performance had been reinforced over many years, and there were numerous poorly performing employees and managers throughout the hospital who had never even been told that their performance was unacceptable, much less been terminated. In contrast to the lack of formal organizational rewards, the paper-scraps admitting system gave the admitting staff power—a significant reward—in that no one else understood how it worked and it was so critical to the hospital. Further, it provided an opportunity to do favors for the physicians, whose thanks, expressed verbally and through gifts, were important and valued rewards for the admitting staff. Therefore, they were quite motivated to retain the peculiar and inefficient system that allowed them to gain many rewards.

A final example is very common in hospitals, where physicians' economic goals do not always coincide with the hospital's. It is generally in the hospital's interest to expand its medical staff and offer admitting privileges to skilled physicians who do not yet practice there, because they will provide additional admissions. Physicians currently on staff see other physicians with similar competencies as competition for referrals and for current patients. Such competition would result in loss of revenue for the established physicians. Therefore, they work hard to maintain control of the process of granting medical staff appointments, and thereby over hospital expansion. Also, physicians are adversely affected economically when they serve in leadership roles or participate in hospital committees or task forces. In a community hospital, each hour that a physician spends on administrative issues takes away from billings and/or from incentives built into his or her medical group practice.

We typically think of rewards in financial terms, but rewards in organizations are not limited to money. They can take the form of increased responsibility, increased control over resources, formal job progression, and acknowledgment from respected people. Especially where little emphasis is placed on setting formal goals and providing rewards to those who meet their goals, people look for acknowledgment from others and for other, more subtle cues about their performance.

Groups have powerful effects on members' behavior, for they can provide or withhold rewards that meet social needs and are an important source of feedback on behavior. Group norms can be supportive of organizational goals or they can be dysfunctional. Rarely are these discussed explicitly. Usually indirectly, and through trial and error, a new member of a group learns its norms. People risk sanctions from their peers for behaving in a way that does not conform to the group's norms. For example, a manager must be careful in taking on "too much" responsibility lest he or she be sanctioned for "power grabbing."

In nine out of ten times that we are called in to "fix" a "stuck" implementation of integrative organizational arrangements, we find that the norms of the senior management team discourage open communication and problem solving. Typically, the implementation of the new organizational arrangements has made the already existing problem within the senior management group intolerable. Almost always the CEO says he or she wants open communication and does not understand why it is not occurring. In fact, we usually find that the norms of the group are "to be polite in conversation," "not to confront others in meetings," and "not to challenge the ideas of the CEO." As a result, people agree to things that all know no one will actually implement. Is it any wonder that these meetings are unproductive? Usually everybody knows the meetings are unproductive, but to group members it seems impossible to do anything about the situation.

The dysfunctional group is indeed difficult to change. Since the group norms discourage confronting any issue, the group never faces the problem of its own dysfunctional behavior or asks how it can be improved. An implicit sanction against the needed confrontation blocks progress. This sanction must be removed, usually by the leader, sometimes with the assistance of an outside consultant. Removing the sanction is not easy, for it has taken years for the belief to develop that confrontation is "not OK." To establish the trust that a member of the group will not be punished for confronting an issue requires discussion, agreement about the problem facing the group and the need to change, risk taking to confront an issue, and support (in other words, reward) for that new behavior.

It also is important to note that many rewards are not controlled by and may not even originate within organizations. The most striking example of this is Rosenberg's (1989) finding that hospital middle managers are more highly focused on personal career advancement than on hospital performance. Consequently, managers seek to achieve outcomes that can clearly be attributed to their own efforts and be recognized as accomplishments by other organizations that potentially might recruit them. Behavior, therefore, is directed at achievable, not too risky, visible outcomes over which an individual manager has substantial control. These typically are departmentally oriented, not hospitalwide or interdepartmental. If Rosenberg's conclusions are valid, then they further highlight the importance of managing the rewards that encourage desired behaviors.

Weisbord (1976) also has noted the strength of the professional identity system and its impact on professionals' behavior in hospitals. Most professionals identify first with their profession and specialization and introduce themselves that way (for example, "I'm a pediatric cardiologist"). Their hospital affiliation is secondary. When physicians regularly admit to several hospitals, how can they have a deep organizational commitment to any one? The strength of professional identification is exemplified by a medical school dean who once told us that if we wanted to interview his faculty, we should schedule to meet them at O'Hare Airport, since half of them were always there changing planes to go to professional meetings. It is little wonder that physicians seem so difficult to control, and it is a fact that forces outside the hospital are significant factors.

In addressing this situation, it is important to recognize that forces external to the organization are important to the professions and to professionals. Denying this is unrealistic. Arguing to professionals that external factors should not be important will have little effect other than to increase their defensiveness and reduce the credibility of anyone arguing that position. Further, it is productive to shift the focus from one of *controlling* to one of *influencing* the behavior of professionals. It is not possible to control. It is possible to influence. Doing so requires making it desirable for physicians and others to change their behavior. This can be accomplished through persuasion and by altering rewards to make it advantageous for people to behave in the desired manner.

Rewards for Integrative Management

When a new organizational structure is being implemented, roles, responsibilities, and power are in an ambiguous state. At such a time, people are especially keen to resolve the ambiguity, and they seek subtle cues from all corners of the organization. (Is it any wonder why the "grapevine" works so well?) It is important to consider and manage the subtle cues as well as the formal ones. For example, a significant subtle cue is given in asking someone to participate in a task force or work group, telling the person you value their contribution, but then scheduling the group's meetings so that the person cannot possibly attend. The real message is transmitted by the action, not by the words.

When integrative arrangements are being implemented, the roles of integrative managers are being added or extended. Always at issue are what the integrative manager's scope of authority and influence is, and how it compares with that of the department managers. It is a time when, despite the fear of change and unwillingness to lose power, department managers need to cooperate with integrative managers. If this cooperation is not reflected in rewards, it is unlikely to happen.

Many integrative managers themselves also are asking what their influence is in the organization. Many cues affect perceived influence. For example, if integrative managers' offices are located in the executive suite, they will be perceived as "executives," with high status and strong influence in the organization. If their offices are in patient care areas, they will be perceived as "operations managers" or "clinical managers," closer to the actual delivery of service and more a part of the clinical activity, but not "executive level." If they are located in a building separate from the hub of activity, they will be perceived as relatively low in status and not truly involved in important operational decisions. Which image is best depends on the form of organization desired to support the organizational strategy.

A Recommended Structure for a System of Formal Rewards

In a hospital there are four levels of rewards that require attention: individual, group, department and integrative program, and total organization (system rewards). Since we want to encourage individual staff and managers to achieve high performance, goal setting and rewards based on individual performance are most helpful in encouraging desired behavior. In fact, the most direct impact on an individual's behavior will be rewards based on the individual's performance. Generally, we also want to encourage teamwork and do not want individuals' efforts to be counterproductive. Integrative arrangements are built to facilitate coordination. They acknowledge the interdependencies among staff. Thus, it is important to use the reward system to encourage cooperative behavior. Therefore, basing some rewards on team accomplishments is important. If this is not done, team efforts may only be given lip service.

In integrative arrangements, attaining a balance between departments and integrative programs is critical. Since each has a different and somewhat inherently conflicting perspective, it is important to reward both and not one to the exclusion of the other. Thus, integrative managers should be rewarded on program performance, and department managers rewarded on departmental performance, but not exclusively. In both cases, performance expectations and rewards should also reflect total organizational performance. Where triads are used, all triad members should receive a significant portion of their rewards based on triad and program performance. Where individuals have dual roles, both their operational responsibilities and their integrative responsibilities should be reflected in their rewards.

We suggest a formal reward system that consists of a goal-setting process and an evaluation based on achievement of those goals. The goals should reflect organizational performance; departmental or integrative program performance, depending upon the manager in question; group (if distinct from department or integrative program) performance; and individual performance. Possible weightings might be 90 percent hospital and 10 percent individual for the chief executive; and 40 percent hospital, 40 percent integrative program or traditional department, and 20 percent individual goals for an integrative manager or department manager. These weightings would encourage a focus on individual goals without excluding organizational goals and outcomes. A special case is a triad of administrative leader, nurse leader, and physician leader all jointly responsible for program performance. This triad might also set goals for its effectiveness and accomplishments together, including group goals in addition to the hospital, program, and individual goals. Appropriate weightings on the four levels of goals might be 30 percent each for hospital, integrative program, and group, and 10 percent for individual goals.

Other Rewards

One of the most critical commodities in an organization is time. How people spend their time, and whether they allow other activities to prevent their involvement in integrative efforts or give them a priority, depends to a great extent on the perceived rewards. By publicly recognizing managers' and staff's integrative efforts and accomplishments, leaders can reward them and indicate the importance of the integrative efforts to the rest of the organization. This can be achieved in meetings, through an organization's newsletter, or even in the community news media. Providing this recognition is an important leadership function. Conversely, if people's efforts are not recognized, the subtle cue is given that they are not important, and the opportunity to enhance motivation is lost. Highlighting integrative efforts indicates a shift in an organization's reward structure. Care should be taken, however, not to undermine departmental efforts. Both in balance are critical to success.

Furthermore, if organizational leaders support behaviors that are inappropriate for integrative approaches, they will undermine the integration. For example, allowing a department or a physician to go around an integrative manager and get a special exception that affects the integrative program encourages the undesired behavior and discredits the integrative manager. In a triad, allowing one member to work behind the scenes against the position of the other two splinters the triad, reduces trust among its members, and renders it ineffective. Although in both cases the rationale for the action may seem very logical and compelling, the act of supporting the behavior is dysfunctional for achieving integration.

Physician involvement is an important objective of integrative arrangements. The structure facilitates involvement of medical leadership, but does not directly achieve that involvement. Integrative program effectiveness is directly affected by the degree of physician commitment and involvement, however. Thus, it is important to consider the rewards to physicians for their involvement. As discussed previously, time is a highly valued commodity for most physicians. They often view leadership responsibilities not as valued positions, but rather as obligations to be met when "it's your turn."

To overcome these costs, or negative rewards, of involvement, other rewards must be developed and promoted. One of the most powerful ones is ensuring that involvement leads to better care for the physician's patients and a better, smoother working environment. Effective integrative arrangements will provide these results, leading to greater intrinsic rewards for physicians practicing there. Being part of a successful effort is also an important reward. Participating in meetings where issues that are important to physicians are addressed effectively and where things are accomplished is rewarding. Other rewards include improved responsiveness from administration, better relationships with nursing and with other physicians and medical specialties, and more say in how things are done. It is critical to win physicians over to integrative arrangements. A good first step is simply to ask them how they would want to make the service function better and to provide access and responsiveness to their legitimate needs.

Organizational Culture

Several of the examples we have given so far refer to aspects of organizational culture (Deal and Kennedy, 1982), although we have not explicitly used that term. Organizational culture is akin to societal culture. It is the accepted way of doing things in an organization—the shared values and the norms. Culture is pervasive in its influence on the behavior of managers, medical staff, and other employees. Culture is affected by but not limited to the formal reward system. It is conveyed formally, through goal setting and discussion of norms, as well as informally, often through stories.

Culture pervades all corners of organizational life and is recognizable to visitors as well as to organizational members. When you first walk into a facility you can make an initial assessment of the amount of pride people take in the organization. It is reflected in the cleanliness of the facility. Do people—from the CEO to the hourly service worker—routinely pick up paper on the floor, or do most people walk right by and say "It's not my job"? We have been in facilities where the pride in the organization has been so strong that we as visitors have picked up discarded paper. We have also been in facilities whose appearance has appalled us.

Just as society's values and norms can be changed, so can an organization's culture. For example, in the United States twenty years ago it was socially acceptable to smoke tobacco, and more meetings were held in smoke-filled rooms than in clean air. Today that has changed dramatically. Similarly, many organizations that have rewarded, even encouraged, such dysfunctional behaviors as treating patients and visitors impolitely have successfully changed their norms and values—and employees' behavior. However, this is not an easy task that can be accomplished with a quick fix. Furthermore, many organizations have attempted various approaches to change and have failed, which reinforces the belief that things will never change. Organizational culture is supported by the history of the organization, by its formal and informal rewards, by the role models set by influential people in the organization, and by what is communicated as being important, tolerated, or unacceptable. Changing a long history of reinforcement of an old culture takes several years of consistent support and reward. Changing attitudes throughout an organization from "We have always done it that way" to "What can I do better?" and "How can we creatively work together to provide better services to patients?" realistically cannot be done in a few months.

Conclusion

The reward system is a crucial element in implementing integrative arrangements. By definition, in implementing innovative structures and practices, behaviors must change. To achieve these changes, the reward system is an important tool. It can be used to encourage desired behavior and focus attention on organizationally desired outcomes, or, if mismanaged, it can encourage dysfunctional behavior.

Most critical to remember in considering the implications of reward systems in health care organizations are these points:

1. Reward desired behavior and use great caution to not inadvertently reward undesired behavior.
2. Use rewards to support the desired balance of influence, gener-

ally to increase integrative managers' influence, and to convey their importance in the organization.

3. Make extrinsic rewards contingent upon performance, and balance performance goals and associated rewards among organizational, integrative program or department, group, and individual levels.

4. Build or refine organizational systems to facilitate people's getting their work done. This will provide them the greatest opportunities for intrinsic rewards.

5. Many subtle things are seen as rewards and/or indications of approval. Manage them.

6. Create and use opportunities for public recognition of integrative efforts and accomplishments.

7. Do not underestimate the impact of organizational culture on individual behavior. Changing the culture may be one of the most important aspects of implementing integrative arrangements. Effecting that change will take a minimum of several years and must start with commitment at the most senior levels of the organization.

8. Do not expect physicians to participate in integrative programs out of generosity or because it is the "right thing" to do. Make it rewarding and beneficial to them.

Chapter Five

Matching Integrative
Structures and
Information Systems

Information is the grist for the decision-making mill. All organizations face the challenge of ensuring that the people responsible for making various decisions have the information they need to make those decisions effectively. With the augmented focus on making program decisions that is characteristic of innovative organizations comes new information requirements. For example, effective decisions to reduce the costs of care can only be made if appropriate information is available on the critical factors that affect costs.

Organizations never have all of the information they need. For example, whether for-profit or not-for-profit, organizations virtually never know all the reasons customers choose their products or services. Although some firms spend considerable sums of money to learn more about consumer preferences, some uncertainty remains in the decision-making process. If industries operated with perfect information, we would not have had the Edsel or New Coke. In the realm of health, however, an even larger gap exists between the information needed to manage organizations and the information available. Larry Weed, M.D., the developer of *The Problem-Oriented*

Medical Record and a commentator on medicine in the United States, notes that "American medicine is like playing darts without a dart board. We play, tossing darts and believing we are right on target. Then someone comes along and puts up the dart board, and we find out we have been far from hitting a bullseye" (Larry Weed, 1973). This situation has been changing as the public in general, the federal government, and the Joint Commission on Accreditation of Healthcare Organizations have increased their focus on outcomes. Nonetheless, this effort still has far to go to provide sufficient assessment of health care organizational performance.

As discussed throughout this book, the traditions of separating clinical and managerial responsibilities and of focusing separately on each profession, department, and specialty have prevented recognition of the needs for information about issues that cross those internal organizational lines. Recognition of the need for this type of information has increased as organizations have considered implementation of integrative approaches.

Historically, clinical and administrative data have been collected, managed, and used independently, reflecting the emphasis on differentiation between clinical and managerial responsibilities. It is foolish, however, to believe that clinical and managerial decisions are totally independent. Management decisions create the context for clinical work (Charns and Schaefer, 1983, chap. 2). For example, decisions on staffing and equipment acquisition directly affect availability of diagnostic and therapeutic procedures. Conversely, clinical decisions have significant impact on financial performance, traditionally viewed as a managerial concern. Clinical decision making could include consideration of financial aspects if appropriate information were available. For example, the costs of medications can be provided to clinicians to assist them in choosing alternatives. Thus, while there are distinct clinical and managerial uses of information, they need to be combined for many purposes, both clinical and managerial. It is most effective, therefore, to collect, aggregate, and report information in a manner that allows clinical and managerial needs to be considered jointly when necessary.

In this chapter we will discuss the fit between organizational arrangements and information systems, and the conceptual design and use of information systems. We also will examine how the pattern of information flow in organizations affects the distribution of power and how information can substantially affect people's attention and motivation. In addition, we will examine some practical issues involving the implementation and use of information systems.

We should note that while the concepts discussed in this chapter do not require a computer, in practice, only a computerized information system is practical for handling the volumes of data involved in healthcare management and for disseminating them in a timely way. As we write this, we know of many hospitals that have allowed the computer revolution to pass them by.

The reader will soon find that this chapter, in comparison to the rest of this book, is more technically oriented. Due to the nature of the concept of information systems in health care, and to their dual clinical and managerial focus, some of the terms used are financially oriented. We want to alert the reader that although the concepts that follow are critical to successful integrative efforts, using these financial terms directly with a clinical audience may be counterproductive. The implementation of integrative efforts must take into consideration language barriers and the varying and sometimes conflicting goals and professional perspectives among the diverse participants. Credibility and trust among the participants must be established and serve as the foundation that allows both financially and clinically oriented constituents to work as a team to enhance the efficiency and effectiveness of care provided to patients.

Fitting an Information System to an Organization

Significant characteristics of the innovative organizations discussed in this book are the placement of decision making at levels of the organization that are close to the point of delivery of service, and the integration of different perspectives in the making of decisions. Until recently, hospital information systems were designed only around the traditional departmental structure, primarily to meet the needs of individual departments and their financial management. For example, hospital budgets and the reporting of actual expenses have included salaries and wages for each department, but have not reflected how efforts of personnel have been utilized to deliver care to particular types of patients, identified by medical condition, source of referral, type of payer, and the like, or to patients of any particular physician or physician group.

The only exceptions to this pattern have occurred when a cost center, or part of the organization for which costs were separately tracked, coincided with a specific type of patient or group of physicians. For example, salaries of nursing staff are typically reported by the area of the hospital to which the staff are assigned, such as floor or patient care unit. For an area such as an intensive care unit, which serves a well-defined group of patients and often (but not always) a limited group of physicians, at least a substantial portion of the costs of caring for those patients could be determined. But this has been the exception, rather than the rule.

Information has been available to manage departments individually, but not to consider many issues that involve two or more departments. For example, if integrative managers wanted to determine whether social workers or nurses could most cost-effectively perform discharge planning for their programs, they would require information on salary expenses for each discipline. Unless there were no differences in the time each discipline required to do discharge planning, time estimates also would be needed. It also would be valuable to see whether a change in discharge planning efforts might affect length of stay, patient satisfaction, or readmission rates. These and other issues of staffing mix and assessment of outcomes are important for integrative managers, who should be concerned with the overall delivery of services in their programs, as well as costs and outcomes.

A traditional hospital information system does not provide the information needed for integrative managers to consider these questions. Usually, only senior management would have access to information from both departments, and that information would not specify efforts required by different types of patients or programs. As a result, they could only make gross comparisons for the total patient population. Thus, the information system would limit the integrative managers' ability to make effective program-focused decisions.

A specialty service in a large hospital provides another example. After years of managing the service piecemeal, the physician service chief, nursing director for the service, and administrative vice president responsible for the service began meeting together on a regular basis as a team to collaboratively manage the service (number 6 on the organizational continuum shown in Figure 2.1). Each manager had a separate budget that was a component of the larger budgets of their respective areas of responsibility. For example, the nursing director's budget was one part of the total nursing department budget. Thus, the three managers had different information about their service, and no comprehensive budget for the whole service existed.

In developing capital equipment budget requests for the upcoming fiscal year, each manager was asked to prioritize items and submit them through departmental channels. As their budgets were aggregated into their departments' total budgets, priorities typically were altered from the perspectives of the different departments. The resulting priorities in the three budgets often were unrelated. This process often led the budget committee to approve items in one budget (for example, the chief's), but not to allow related items in one or both of the other budgets (those of the vice president and nursing director). Recognizing that this did not contribute to the efficient management of the specialty service, the three managers developed a single composite budget request. To do this, they had to go around the budget system, rather than use it to assist them. The hospital's management information system, and in particular its budgeting process, hindered rather than supported the integrative management approach. Recognizing this limitation, the hospital began a revised capital equipment budgeting process. Without revising the process and similarly changing the operating budget and reporting system, the hospital could not achieve the integrative management objectives it sought.

With the implementation of innovative, integrative arrangements, people are asked to determine not only the cost of care for particular types of cases but also patient satisfaction and even efficacy, and they are stifled in their efforts by the lack of information available to them. Innovative organizational forms require integrative managers to be knowledgeable and influential—if not specifically responsible—for some or all of the following regarding their programs: clinical quality, patient satisfaction, staff satisfaction, productivity, utilization, financial performance, planning, and marketing.

Since most hospital information systems were built to support a traditional departmental structure at a time when other ways of managing were not even considered, it should be no surprise that these systems are unable even to capture data in a form that allows integrative reports by program. In fact, many of these systems do not do a very good job of reporting information by department, for many were built primarily for external aggregate organization financial reporting and not for internal management control purposes. This leaves the organization that has implemented an innovative structure in the awkward situation of asking its integrative managers to manage without knowing how they are doing, and therefore with no way of knowing the effectiveness of alternative actions. Nor do they have relevant data to use to persuade others to change or contribute to their programs in different ways. Generally, this leads not only to ineffectiveness but also to frustration.

Lack of information also impairs personnel evaluation, rewards, and feedback. As discussed in the previous chapter, it is very effective to set goals for individuals and base evaluations and rewards on achievement of those goals. For example, some integrative managers have goals of increased market share. Without information on market share, it is not possible to measure performance objectively.

Many hospitals with integrative programs have set program volume goals in terms of diagnosis-related groups (DRGs). Typically, discharge information is available by DRG, but for many programs a DRG may not correspond to a large portion of what an integrative manager does. For example, in one hospital we found that over half of the cardiology admissions were accounted for by physicians other than cardiologists, but cardiologists were the only physicians who worked with the cardiology program manager. Thus, the actual efforts of the program manager had a limited relationship to what was being measured. As this and earlier examples illustrate, care must be taken in implementing integrative management approaches to ensure that essential information is available.

Collection and Dissemination of Information

In designing or considering purchase of an information system there are three major areas in addition to technical issues to consider: what information to collect, how to collect it, and how to aggregate and report it. This process must be driven by a clear determination of the information needs. Data are abundant in health care organizations. What items of data to collect and how to report them depend on the desired uses. Many different aggregations are possible, but only if appropriate identifying information is captured to allow that aggregation. It usually is too late or too costly to capture data after the fact. Thus, for example, discharge diagnosis is commonly available, and it therefore is possible to break down and report various data in terms of individual diagnosis or aggregations of diagnoses, such as by DRGs. This would be adequate for monitoring various performance indicators by DRG. However, if DRGs and integrative programs do not correspond, and it is desired to manage by program, then it is important to ask how data are to be coded to capture program designation. If this is left until after the fact, it may no longer be possible to collect the needed information.

The second issue to consider is how to collect needed data. It is important to remember that costs are incurred in collecting data, and that the costs need to be managed. Therefore, it is best that data be collected once and used for different purposes. Also, it is foolhardy to assume that professionals will willingly provide and enter or transcribe information if they do not see doing so as beneficial to themselves, their practice, or their patients. Thus, expecting that physicians or nurses will enter data that are needed for management reporting purposes but that have little or no clinical value is unrealistic. It is better to build the collection of managerial data into the clinical data management process than to expect people to make additional efforts to provide it.

The final issue to consider is the aggregation of information into usable measures. It is important to remember to plan not only for today's uses of the information but also for the future's. Most computerized information systems (unless they are severely limited) allow reformatting of information with relative ease, thus accommodating even unforeseen future needs. The more critical factor, then, is ensuring that the appropriate identifying information be collected to allow aggregations by whatever basis is needed, now or later.

The Cost and Value of Information

As part of the design of data acquisition, it is critical to determine the value of information and to balance that against the cost of collecting it. Integrative program managers typically have responsibility for cost of services delivered in their programs. Therefore, they need information on the costs and the volume of different services their programs utilize. For example, it is important to know the cost of laboratory procedures. In fact, it probably is important to know the different costs of different laboratory procedures. Making this distinction—between laboratory procedures in general and specific laboratory procedures—increases the cost of obtaining the desired information. In the former case it would be sufficient to sum total labor, supplies, and other costs and divide by the total number of tests performed by the clinical laboratories. Although actual expenses and volume data are used, this approach yields the mean cost of all tests as an estimate of each test. Some tests actually are more expensive and some less. To determine where and how changes could be made in their programs' utilization of laboratory services, integrative managers often need more precise information than such estimates provide. Using averages to estimate costs can cause integrative managers to make improper decisions.

Very precise information can be obtained through microcosting. This process involves directly measuring the time taken to complete a specific process, such as a test, and the supplies and materials consumed. Typically, this measurement is performed by an industrial engineer. Since it is very time consuming to perform microcosting, it is more expensive than merely averaging the costs of an array of procedures. Given the thousands of procedures and processes that are performed in a hospital, it is impossible to perform microcosting on all.

Other estimating procedures offer alternatives to microcosting and to using average departmental costs. For example, one compromise approach to using the average for a whole department is to estimate costs by section of the department. Another approach is to have the most informed managers estimate the costs of different tests, based on their experience. Alternatively, they may estimate the ratios between the costs of different tests. By knowing the average cost of all tests, the ratios can be used to calculate estimates of the cost of each type of test.

In determining whether gross estimates, more focused estimates, averages, or microcosting should be employed to determine the cost of any procedure or service, it is important to weigh the costs of obtaining information against the value of having more accurate information. A key question to ask is whether any decisions or actions would differ substantially, depending on the precision of the information. Other issues to consider are the importance of the decision, the potential impact of variation in elements of cost to be considered, the volume of the procedure in question, and the magnitude of its cost. It would be unwise to expend considerable management time and energy or thousands of dollars to measure actual costs when such efforts could lead to saving only a few hundred dollars.

Cost-to-Charge Ratios

Since management of program costs and use of cost information in program planning are often the focus of integrative managers, it is important to examine one other widely used approach to estimating costs: cost-to-charge ratios. These ratios have been used widely in the health care industry because charges for each test and procedure are known, and a convenient and inexpensive estimate of cost can be obtained by multiplying a cost-to-charge ratio by the charge. Although over a large number of items in an institution the average cost-to-charge ratio might be a stable measure, for individual items the ratio can vary substantially and mask important differences among departments and among specific items. For example, in one hospital we found that from one year to the next the cost-to-charge ratios for certain departments fluctuated by more than 100 percent, and managers had no understanding of the causes of these variations. This hospital obtained cost information from its general ledger, and could account for costs only to the level of individual departments. Program managers relied on this information to project the impact of increasing volume of services, but the accuracy of their projections was limited by the unexplained high variation in cost-to-charge ratios and the lack of other, more direct, measures of actual costs.

This hospital's financial system was developed prior to the mid 1980s. At that time, before the introduction of prospective payment and fixed price contracts for services provided to HMOs, there were few if any incentives to manage costs carefully. Costs were reimbursed based on the institution's total expenses. However, as the need to manage costs increased, so did the importance of obtaining accurate information about the costs of individual procedures. When the hospital implemented integrative program management using direct contact (number 3 on the organizational continuum shown in Figure 2.1) and attempted to plan for new services, it found it lacked necessary information to plan effectively.

Although a rough approximation of a department's costs might be derived from its charges, there is no reason to assume that the ratio of charges to actual costs for any one department is the same as for other departments. This assumption is implicit in the use of institutionwide cost-to-charge ratios, since the estimated cost for a procedure in any one department is based on the charge for that procedure multiplied by the institution's overall average cost-to-charge ratio. Thus, this estimation of costs does not at all reflect a department's actual expenses.

If expenses are aggregated for each department and departmental charges also are aggregated, then cost-to-charge ratios can be calculated for each department individually. Some organizations then use these departmental cost-to-charge ratios to determine the costs of individual procedures within departments. Although better than a single institutional cost-to-charge ratio, departmental cost-to-charge ratios are also limited in their application, for they are based on the implicit assumption that the cost-to-charge ratio is invariate for different procedures within a department. This assumption may not be valid. In determining whether finer aggregations of information are needed, the considerations for use of microcosting, discussed above, again should be applied.

Timeliness of Information

Critical among the attributes that make information valuable is timeliness. If information is not accessible when it is needed to make a decision, it is of little value. For example, if laboratory test results are not available when a physician is making a diagnosis, they are of no use in determining the course of treatment. Except for confirmatory purposes and to support a course of action in case it is questioned after the fact, the lab tests whose results are not available in a timely manner are a waste of resources.

In one major hospital we studied only a few years ago, routine laboratory results were available only twice a day. They were transcribed into a log, then medical students copied them and carried them to the patients' charts. Decisions based on lab work were held up until the results were made available, which delayed treatment and increased patients' length of stay. To say the least, the delivery of information was not timely, and this factor had a substantial negative impact on patient care.

The importance of timeliness is not restricted to clinical information. Organizations often produce internal financial reports on a monthly basis, and these may only be available several weeks after the month being reported, or even later. This information comes too late to be useful for taking corrective action—for example, to bring expenses into line with budget. Several weeks of spending typically occur before the information is available, to alert managers to the problem and allow them to initiate changes. Faced with the lack of needed information from the organization, effective managers often keep their own records to track spending in their areas. They then monitor the information in the organization's budget reports to make sure the accounting department "got it right." These efforts, of course, are duplicative, but they may be seen by the manager as necessary in order to provide critical information in a timely manner when the organizational systems do not do so.

Historically, computer systems have operated in a "batch" mode, with financial reports produced on a regular cycle, such as monthly. When delays occur in entering information into the system, revenues or expenses may easily be omitted from reports. This could result in erroneous conclusions about the financial situation.

Advancements in computer systems have made it possible to obtain on-line reports upon request. However, unless information is captured on-line when expenses are encumbered and revenues earned, or unless they at least are entered in a timely manner, the resulting reports will still not reflect the actual situation and may lead to inappropriate decisions. Since increased organizational responsiveness and empowerment of integrative managers are objectives of most integrative organization redesigns, availability of timely information should be a particular concern.

Intermediate Products

Although conceptually we might argue that it has always been important to manage not only individual departments but also their combined outputs in providing care during episodes of illness (or longer), health care organizations have not done so. Innovative, integrative organizations bring this need into sharp focus.

No matter what the organization structure, an individual department rarely provides the total service that any patient needs. For example, the clinical laboratories typically do not perform a complete blood count (CBC) for a patient independent of other diagnostic and therapeutic interventions directed at relieving a specific health problem. Thus, we should not view a CBC or any other diagnostic procedure as a product, or output, of a hospital. Rather, diagnostic and therapeutic interventions are part of a larger service delivered to a patient, and it is the larger, overall service that is a hospital's true output.

The CBC, while not a *final product,* is a product resulting from a combination of inputs in the forms of labor, materials, and capital equipment. Conceptually, then, we can see the CBC as an *intermediate product.* Inputs are combined to produce intermediate products, which in turn are combined to produce the final products or services, which are the ultimate outputs of the organization (see Figure 5.1).

Each traditional hospital department produces a host of intermediate products. In addition to CBCs, the clinical laboratories produce intermediate products ranging from lead screening to bacterial cultures. Similarly, the radiology department produces a

Figure 5.1. Intermediate Products Contribute to Total Output.

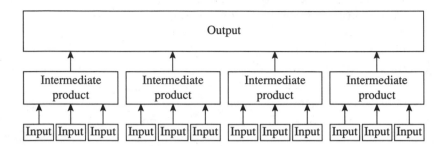

number of diagnostic and therapeutic intermediate products, from routine chest X-rays to radiation therapy treatments. Although traditionally not viewed as such, a day of nursing care at a particular level of intensity is also an intermediate product.

Using the concept of intermediate products helps to distinguish responsibilities and manage relationships between departments and integrative programs. The departments have primary responsibility for the costs and quality of intermediate products, which result from their efficient and effective combination of the organization's inputs. The integrative programs are responsible for combining intermediate products into final products. The volume of intermediate products used and the quality of final products are thus the responsibility of the integrative programs. Departments have little direct contact with nurses or physicians who order and use their intermediate products; it is difficult, therefore, for departments to control the volume or appropriate use of these products.

Although integrative managers do not have complete control over utilization, they are in a position to influence utilization of intermediate products in several ways. First, through personal persuasion and feedback of utilization information, they may directly influence physicians' decisions. Second, in organizational configurations where they have greater influence and responsibility, integrative managers can affect the care delivery process through their decisions on staffing and other resources, by helping clinicians coordinate their efforts to work together more effectively and efficiently, and by improving systems, removing barriers and inefficiencies, and solving problems that affect the delivery process.

Given the distinction between final products and intermediate products, it is appropriate and helpful to use the cost and quality of a department's intermediate products as measures of its performance. These measures can include integrative groups' satisfaction with those services, their responsiveness and timeliness, and patients' satisfaction with the services delivered. Integrative managers are more appropriately assessed on the overall functioning of their programs. Recognizing that they lack complete control but can have some influence over use of intermediate products, it is also helpful to link integrative managers' goals to volume of intermediate products utilized and to use this as one evaluative measure of their performance.

Some departments are responsible for both intermediate and final products. For example, we have argued that the nursing department should participate in managing integrative teams and task forces. In such positions, nurse managers are responsible for both intermediate products in their nurse manager roles and final products in their integrative roles. Even for a manager with dual roles, using the concept of intermediate product helps clarify departmental and integrative responsibilities. Throughout a hospital organization, this concept can address many relationships between departments and integrative groups and help clarify responsibilities and measurement.

The concept of intermediate product also provides a way for integrative managers to discuss with departments the specifications and characteristics of services they provide. For example, integrative managers and the director of the clinical laboratories can discuss response times and differences in cost for standard and stat tests. If there are no differences in cost to the program, management and staff in the program have little incentive to avoid stat tests. However, if the program is charged differently for stat and regular requests, an incentive is provided to request stat tests only when they actually are needed. Although the financial implications typically are appreciated most by the integrative managers, explicit information is available with this approach to convey to staff in the program. As clinicians become more conscious of the cost of care and their impact on it, they will perceive greater importance in this information.

To continue with the example of the clinical laboratories, their performance also can be assessed against the agreed upon response time for routine and stat tests. This can be used as a basis for discussing any proposed changes, whether suggested by the integrative program or the clinical laboratories.

While to some readers this approach may seem overly explicit, it provides relevant information for scheduling, and it facilitates planning by reducing the number of unknown factors typically present in managing a program. Further, it not only helps establish departmental performance standards but also provides a basis for measuring managerial performance that is more closely aligned to the reality of responsibilities than traditional systems allow. Additionally, this approach can be used to facilitate collaboration among integrative managers and departmental managers in determining the implications of changes in departments' volume and costs that are driven by an integrative program.

Since hospitals have traditionally categorized information only in terms of the inputs utilized, information on the outputs of the organization, on intermediate products, and on the relationship among these three have not been available. Thus, most hospitals must implement new information systems in order to reap the benefits of their integrative organizations.

One last item to consider is that most hospitals have a number of information systems that were designed for special uses. Examples are laboratory systems, patient acuity systems, financial systems, personnel systems, and the like. Unfortunately, these systems are often unable to communicate with each other effectively. The isolated pockets of information they contribute are of less value than integrated information from the various systems would be. Remedying these problems may require systems hardware and software modifications, and if common identifying data are not contained in the different systems, more radical redesigns will need to be implemented.

Matching Organization Design to an Information System

In contrast to the situations already discussed, some hospitals have approached innovation by implementing new information systems first; but then they are unable to utilize their capabilities because they lack appropriate organizational arrangements. In these situations the information system is a more powerful tool than the organization can utilize; in the situations discussed previously, the information system's inadequacies limited the effectiveness of the organization design. Both cases represent a mismatch between the organization design and the information system. Higher performance could be achieved by improving one to match the capabilities of the other.

In reality, no organization should be designed solely to meet the requirements of its information system. However, because they have not had appropriate organization designs and management practices, many hospitals have been disappointed with the limited impact of the new, sophisticated information systems that they have installed. Although the new systems do provide information needed for managing programs, the organization has not empowered or even designated anyone to act on that information. Unless capable integrative managers are in place, with responsibility for managing programs, the information available from the system cannot be used to improve organizational performance. An information system and an organization structure must complement each other, with the choice of both information system and structure following from an organization's strategy.

If an organization intends a limited use of program information, a limited integrative structure is sufficient. For example, if the information is to be used to affect the behavior of groups of physicians, then utilizing direct contact is sufficient (number 3 on the structural continuum, Figure 2.1). In this case, different integrative managers work with different physician groups—for example, by specialty. Program managers can review information on admissions and utilization and, through direct contact, influence physicians' actions. If, however, a greater impact is desired, involving multiple disciplines collaborating to evaluate and change the delivery of services, stronger integrative mechanisms are needed. Since many decisions in health care require inputs from numerous people or parts of the organization, program information can be used most effectively when the organization brings these people together and encourages and supports their joint decision making.

Just because information is available somewhere in an organization does not mean it will be used effectively. The degree to which program information can be used effectively varies directly with organizational form. The ability to use program information increases along the structural continuum from the pure functional form (number 1) through the matrix form (number 7). Beyond the matrix form to the program organization forms (numbers 8 and 9), the organization's capacity to use program information is not increased, except that division managers have more power than integrative managers in other organizational forms and program information is easier to track in the program organization forms.

In addition to considering organizational form, it is important to recognize the importance of management practices in affecting how information is used. Since people can easily become overloaded with information, they screen out information that does not appear highly relevant. Furthermore, a natural defense mechanism that we all employ is to screen out information incongruent with our current beliefs. Thus, it is important not only to *provide* information needed for management, but also to *organize* to bring together the people who can act on that information, *support* and *empower* them, and *hold them accountable* for using the information in making decisions and taking actions that will make a difference.

Motivational Effects of Information

When people are given meaningful information, it focuses their attention and efforts. This has both desirable and undesirable consequences. As discussed in Chapter Four, focusing people's attention, especially when they have high achievement needs, can direct their efforts toward issues that are being measured. This also means that other issues are given relatively less attention, even to the point of being ignored. A narrowing of focus is almost inevitable because all individuals have cognitive limits. We can handle only so many items of information at once. When presented with more information than we can process, we may become anxious and ultimately ignore some of the information we are getting.

For example, in making a major purchase, we can only keep

track of a limited number of features of a few alternative choices. We cannot focus on all features of all choices. Instead, we rely upon decision-making strategies, such as prioritizing the importance of different features. In buying a new car, for example, most people have difficulty comparing all the options offered by different manufacturers. Once consumers decide to buy a basic model, car salespeople can more easily sell them options because they are no longer comparing the price of the car in question with other manufacturers' models.

In organizations, our inability to focus on all available information has significant impact. If managers are given information on their expenses but not on their revenues, they focus on keeping expenses low, even if doing so results in loss of revenue that would exceed the savings. If volume of procedures is reported but not total revenue, people who get that information will focus on increasing volume, even if efforts could be better placed to increase total revenue. Similarly, if people receive information only on volume or revenues, they will not be attentive to the cost of providing services. If integrative managers are given information only on performance of their programs and not the total organization, their individual program focus will be reinforced. This will discourage cooperation among program managers. In summary, the key issue is that the information people receive contributes substantially to their perceptions of what is important, what is not, and where to direct their attention and efforts.

One example of an organization that recognized these effects and attempted to minimize their negative impacts was a major hospital that was implementing a computerized patient management system. The new system would present activities and a timeline for their completion, based on a patient's condition. The system design group, consisting of information systems staff and professionals from several disciplines, recognized that different professionals typically focused only on patient information from their own professions. Physicians, for example, rarely read nurses' notes in the medical record. In developing the system, the design team initially considered having the computer display only those activities traditionally performed by whatever discipline was using the system at the time. For example, a nurse would be shown only "nursing activities.'' The designers recognized, however, that presenting the information in this manner would reinforce the traditional ways of thinking about who actually could perform the various activities. As a result, they agreed to display information on all of the activities to be performed, without regard to who traditionally performed them.

In summary, simply measuring and reporting particular items affects people's focus of attention and motivation. If organizational rewards are related to achievement of measurable items, the effects of the information on motivation are amplified.

Information and Power

The distribution of information in organizations has important implications for the acquisition and use of power. In general, having control over any resource critical to an organization is a source of power. For example, physicians' control over admission of patients, coupled with hospitals' dependence on patient admissions, is a key source of medical staff power. Similarly, information is a resource to an organization, so information is a source of power. The more an organization needs a particular type of information, the more power the source of that information has over others who need that information. Furthermore, the fewer the alternative sources of that information, the greater the power of the sources that do exist.

Often information is available inside or outside an organization, but it must be interpreted to be useful. The people who know how to interpret the information can use their ability as a source of power, since the organization depends on them to provide the information in a usable form. Access to specialized sources of information is also a source of power.

In innovative organizational forms, integrative managers are often in unique positions of having access to information regarding services provided and being able to interpret it. If an integrative manager does not use the information in a coercive manner, it can be an important source of power. The integrative manager's interpretation can also be viewed as a valuable contribution, which in turn will contribute to the manager's perceived competence. In contrast, if performance information is available only for departments and not for programs, integrative managers will be limited in their ability to influence decisions regarding costs or shifts in resources.

Another aspect of the relationship between information and power involves disseminating or withholding information on issues such as financial performance. This is best illustrated through an example. Some programs and specialties have higher earning potential than others. Most people recognize that surgery and surgical subspecialties generate more revenue than primary care specialties, such as pediatrics and family medicine. If the actual hospital revenues attributable to the high-earning departments were made known, this would enhance these departments' power. That would make it more difficult for hospital senior management to allocate resources across specialties in ways that maximized hospitalwide priorities, for the high earners would have information to support arguments for greater expenditures in their areas. This information could not be refuted, and it would focus attention on the high earners. But such information is a simplification of reality. It does not account for the interdependence among programs or the role of traditionally low-earning primary care specialties in providing referrals to other specialties. Contributing to an enhancement of the power of high earners and a diminution of the power of primary care specialties would skew the balance needed among specialties to achieve long-term effectiveness.

Conclusion

Information systems are a powerful clinical and managerial tool. In this chapter we have focused on managerial applications of information systems and the match between organization structure and information systems' capabilities. In implementing innovative organizational arrangements, it is necessary to provide the information that people need to carry out their responsibilities. While this may appear obvious, in most hospitals there is a large gap between the information that is needed and the information that is available. In implementing an information system, it is important to evaluate the need for various items of information, the cost of collecting the information, the value associated with various levels of estimation versus actual measurement, and the timeliness of information availability.

Where a sophisticated information system that allows for integrative decision making has already been implemented, it is important to ensure that the organization structure, responsibilities, support, and rewards allow and encourage its appropriate use. The information system can be compared to the structural alternatives presented in Chapter Two to assess the congruence between the two.

Information has a significant impact on both individual behavior and distribution of power. What, how, and to whom information is disseminated has both desired and undesired consequences. It is preferable to anticipate these consequences and implement a system to support behaviors that are desired and a balanced distribution of power. Assessment of information flows can also reveal where changes need to be made in existing systems.

In closing, we offer the following recommendations, drawn from the concepts presented in this chapter:

1. Ensure that information systems' capabilities meet organizational requirements. The advantages of integrative structures can be limited severely by lack of information needed to make program decisions and evaluate program performance.
2. Conversely, the value of a sophisticated information system is limited by an organization's capability to use it. Choose a structure that has sufficiently powerful integrative capacity and staff it with integrative managers who are able to use the program information.
3. Be careful in using cost estimates. Average costs and cost-to-charge ratios are not actual costs. Use of these and other estimates can lead to erroneous decisions.
4. Balance the cost of obtaining information against the value of that information. When considering direct measurement of costs and microcosting, assess whether the volume, magnitude, or variance in the cost justifies a greater expenditure to obtain more precise measures.
5. Departments should be responsible for the cost and quality of intermediate products, and programs should be responsible for

volume and quality of final products and volume of intermediate products used.

6. Information focuses people's efforts on the items reported.
    Reinforce the desired focus, using caution not to encourage
    unintended and undesired behavior, such as a narrow focus that
    discourages collaboration.

7. Information also affects distribution of power. Manage infor-
    mation dissemination to ensure a balance of power that
    matches organizational needs.

Chapter Six

Implementing
(and Surviving)
the Change Process

The success of an integrative organizational approach depends to a great extent on how it is introduced and implemented in an organization. Inherent in integrative management are shifts in responsibilities and power, new relationships and expectations, new sources of information and measurement, and a new vision for the organization. It presents opportunities for empowerment of staff, but also a challenge to the traditional ways of doing things. How extensive a change is depends on the organizational form that is chosen to be implemented. At a minimum, integrative managers must gain credibility and influence, and department managers must cooperate even when they feel they are losing some control. If task forces (number 4 on the organizational continuum, Figure 2.1) or teams (number 6) are implemented, then more people are involved and the change is more extensive than implementing single integrative managers using direct contact (number 3). Thus, more attention must be given to the process of implementing the change. Similarly, if an organization has a history of resistance to change or unsuccessful attempts to change, more attention and effort are required in the change process. Even in its more limited forms, such as direct contact, however, integrative management is a significant change for an organization. Its effects on members of the organization, and in turn, their impact on the success of the change, should not be underestimated.

As many individuals have learned through experience, there are many ways of saying the same thing in order to bring about a change in an individual's behavior. Blunt statements or orders may get the message across to the recipient but leave such by-products as hurt and resentment. Other approaches will get the same message across to the individual but without the negative by-products. Indeed, when a message is couched in positive terms, the by-products may be appreciation and an unexpected level of commitment to the behavioral change being requested. The same dynamics can be seen in attempts to change the behavior of an organization.

When we compare change management for individuals and for organizations, we can identify some changes that must happen immediately to prevent grave circumstances from occurring. The child who runs across the street without looking needs to be confronted in such a way that immediate change results, regardless of the child's understanding and acceptance of the need for the change. Similarly, an organization that is losing thousands of dollars a day and jeopardizing its future by providing a particular service may need to eliminate the service immediately, without taking the time to allow an alternative to evolve that would be more acceptable to the institution or to the customers of the service.

In contrast, individuals whose diet is not properly balanced have the luxury of some time in order to learn how to improve their diet and modify related behaviors to maintain healthy food habits for the remainder of their lifetimes. They may also be able to share their newfound knowledge and behaviors with family members, and thus the change in life-style initiated by one individual may eventually affect a whole family. The institution that is functioning successfully, but needs to look for a "better way to build a mousetrap" in the future, can take the time and steps necessary to understand the impact that the new "mousetrap production line" will have on operations, finance, and even the individuals involved. In fact, the mousetrap senior management may recognize the value of taking extra time to get employees at all levels involved in the analysis.

Changing an individual or an organization is a complicated process, with aspects that are physical, cultural, and emotional. To bring about a change effectively, these factors need to be recognized and understood and a strategy needs to be developed to prevent, or at least to respond to, any negative consequences of the change. Since implementing an integrative organizational structure often requires substantial modifications to systems, procedures, and culture, it is important to recognize and understand the impact of the change process itself. Therefore, this chapter will describe aspects of organizational change in general, including the typical stages of change, and techniques of facilitating the change process. Additionally, it will relate these concepts to the implementation of integrative organizational forms.

Conventional Wisdom on Change

Although the concept of change is easily regarded as a positive event, in practice, change is often seen and felt as threatening by those it affects. An individual who has recognized the need for a new job can easily see the benefits of such a change. More money, more stature, easier commute—the benefits are easy to recognize. However, when the actual day comes for the person to leave his or her old office, desk, and routine, the comfort of the known is replaced by anxiety about the unknown: Will I succeed? How will I be perceived? Can I really do this new job?

Organizational change is much more than redrawing an organizational chart. It is not only the alteration of procedures, systems, and formal accountabilities but also the reorienting of people's behavior. As an organization and thus its individual members experience change, a whole host of feelings arise. People may be frustrated, frightened, or inspired. New skills may be needed. Managers may have to formulate new philosophies in order to lead the institution differently than they have in the past. Changes in power may result. People in a department that once had power in the organization may feel it slipping away. Staff may feel a loss of control when they are reassigned, new rules are written, budgeting processes are revised, and expectations are changed. For all of these and many more reasons, change is often resisted by individuals—and thus by organizations. It may not be overstating the point to presume that resistance to change is a somewhat instinctual behavior on the part of human beings. There are ways, however, to minimize that resistance. Participative management techniques are among the most important methods for overcoming resistance to change and gaining commitment.

Much of the resistance to integrative organizational forms is predictable. In these new organizational arrangements, shifts in power are inevitable. Department managers will lose some degree of direct control, with the amount of the loss depending on the structural form being implemented, while integrative managers gain power and influence. The change process must support those losing power and engage them in ensuring the success of the change, but it must also make clear and reinforce the roles of integrative managers. Making the change process participative, as will be discussed in greater detail later in the chapter, is one key to successfully managing resistance.

Organizational Culture

Change is a cultural phenomenon. An organization's acceptance of change is indicative of the organization's culture. Some cultures promote change as a desirable state, and thus individuals seek to bring about change. People respond positively to challenges associated with stretching their skills to implement new approaches. They expect and often look forward to being moved out of the "comfort zone," characteristic of the old way of doing things. In this type of culture, the organization and thus individuals' tolerance for change and the ambiguity that accompanies it are greater than in an organization that does not promote change. In the culture of this kind of organization, old habits die hard and the infamous phrase "because we have always done it that way" is accepted as the legitimate reason why things could not happen differently, even if they would be better.

In organizations that do not value and promote change, potentially beneficial changes are also often blocked by the syndrome of "paralysis by analysis." People never feel they have enough information to move ahead with a change, and instead need to wait to study the issue further. In such a situation, it is common to find that the recommendations of one committee studying an issue are followed by the formation of another committee to do further study. All too often, all of the committee reports end up in a file drawer or on a shelf and are never acted upon. This lack of action contributes to future expectations that committee, task force, or team work is not valued, and people avoid involvement or make only minimal effort. In contrast, in a culture where change is promoted, it is likely that making mistakes and learning the hard way are the accepted way of functioning. In the extreme, such organizations are impulsive and initiate change without examining the alternatives or planning sufficiently. They seem to follow the steps "Ready—Fire—Aim," or even "Fire—Ready—Aim."

In the middle of this continuum are cultures that encourage well-thought-out change. Their change process is slower and more deliberate than that of an impulsive organization, but it continually moves forward, as the steps along the way are carefully planned, executed, assessed, and refined. In contrast to organizations that limit change, balanced organizations do analyze and plan, but do not allow excessive analysis to block all implementation. People recognize the value of planning and assessment, but also recognize that ambiguity and uncertainty are inherent in change and that at some point it is necessary to get on with it, even though they cannot predict every last detail of what is going to happen.

The balanced organization expects and prepares for ambiguity. A simple but important step is to admit to the strong—if not inevitable—potential for ambiguity. The leaders of a change effort should admit at the outset that they do not know all the answers and cannot predict all the implications and outcomes, but that the organization has the skills and the desire to learn to cope with the unknown.

Indeed, coping with the unknown is key to an organization's future success. When most organizations enter into new realms, there is a tendency to try to determine, anticipate, and prepare for each and every contingency. When this occurs, there is a strong potential for "paralysis by analysis" to result. Individuals and organizations need to set limits on how much analysis they will do and then admit that other things may happen. And, when they do happen, the organization will swiftly assess the impact and respond as appropriate. Individuals who can accept the fact that there will be unanticipated results are not surprised, and they do not see unanticipated results as symbols of failure when they occur. Rather, unforeseen results are recognized as evidence of the predicted ambiguity. Furthermore, the organizations that effectively manage change learn from unexpected outcomes and are able to predict and handle them better in the future.

Integrative managers, especially, must be able to tolerate ambiguity, for their jobs are not fully defined and they are not given complete control over their areas of responsibility. It is important to recognize that the greatest ambiguity is at the first stages of implementing new integrative positions, when the roles are least well defined and the impacts on other departments are not completely known. Searching for formal authority at these times is not the answer. Working collaboratively, showing others the benefits their participation will bring, and achieving valued results from the change are key steps in implementing the new positions and managing the ambiguity. Senior managers' recognition of the inherent ambiguity, their reassurance and reiteration of the vision for change, and their support of the integrative managers are critical.

The Systems Nature of Organizations

Is it possible to change just one thing? We would suggest that the answer is a flat no. One small change may actually be the first "domino" in a long line of changes. Some of these secondary results can be identified and planned for. As for others, the interdependence of issues may be difficult to detect and thus may not be foreseeable. However, a good rule of thumb is to remember that organizations are complex and interdependent systems. A change in any one area typically affects many others, and thus it is important to consider the potential implications of a change.

Hospitals are among the most complex and interdependent of all organizations. As a result, it is more likely than in other types of organizations that a change in one part will affect many of its other components. For example, one hospital wanted to develop a chest pain center and to streamline admissions for patients with chest pain. In studying the admission of a typical patient presenting with chest pain, the hospital noted the involvement of private physicians, house staff, the emergency department, the admitting department, general medical floors, the escort service, and laboratories, as well as the cardiac care unit and other parts of cardiology. It was not possible to change the admitting process just for patients with chest pain without changing many parts of the system other than cardiology.

Another, more general example occurs when people focus on improving the content of one job or set of jobs; they will commonly forget that changes in those jobs will affect the responsibilities and possibly the skills required of the jobs' supervisor. Many organizations have attempted to improve jobs and increase their inherent motivation by empowering the employees who hold those jobs and giving them greater responsibilities. Often where these efforts have failed, no one has recognized supervisors and helped them develop new skills and prepare for their employees' having greater responsibilities. It is not unusual for the supervisors to wonder what is left for them to do if their employees have more responsibility. In fact, they may be threatened by the change. In such cases, the supervisors will not support the change and may actively subvert it.

Finally, replacing even one employee in an organization is a change that will most likely cause reverberations well beyond that one job. The new individual may have different strengths and limitations than the former employee. As a result, other individuals' jobs may be affected. The new employee also may develop a different routine from the former one, thus requiring others to adapt their routines.

Pace of Change: Evolution or Revolution?

Evolution or revolution . . . what kind of change would you like to see occur? With most change that is not emergent in nature, this question needs to be answered, and it dictates the strategy for change. We would advocate for the evolutionary process, for a multitude of reasons. First, evolution allows individuals to grow, learn new skills, and develop the trust and new relationships that are needed in any new organizational form. Additionally, an evolutionary approach allows time to develop and implement the new methods and systems that are required. Second, problems and shortfalls can be anticipated and detected more easily, so that solutions can be developed before a state of crisis develops. Third, the loss felt for the old way of life is less severe because individuals have time to adapt and reflect on the benefits of the new rather than holding tightly to the old way in order not to be forced suddenly into the unknown. Fourth, evolution provides the time for people to participate actively in creating the new ways of working, thereby reducing resistance to the change. Finally, change that takes the form of adaptation can occur in a natural progression, unlike an urgently designed and implemented new system. Natural cycles in the organization's methods of doing business, such as in its budgeting process, can be utilized to reinforce the changes being adopted. In fact, as discussed in Chapter Four, many people wait to see whether proposed changes will really happen by noting whether the changes are reflected in processes such as budgeting, goal setting, and personnel evaluation. If the new desired behaviors are not reinforced through these organizational processes, people infer that it is "business as usual" and change is not really desired.

Evolution generally is preferred over revolution. However, it is essential not to mire down in a change process that is so slow that no momentum is gained and change does not occur at all. There also are times when revolution is needed. These typically are characterized either by urgency in addressing an issue that cannot be allowed to persist or by an intransigence in the organization that cannot be moved by a slow and deliberate process. We believe that these situations are clearly evident in the critical nature of the issues being addressed.

Senge (1990a) explained the process of implementing change with an analogy to boiling a frog. If you put a frog in a pot of cold water and slowly heat it on the stove, the frog may never notice the heat. Before long, the frog will be cooked! In contrast, if the frog is placed directly into boiling water, it will immediately react by jumping out of the pot to safety. In organizations, effecting a sudden change is sometimes the only means of signaling that the status quo is no longer appropriate or acceptable. However, just as the frog who jumps to safety will avoid in the future anything that looks like boiling water, so may members of an organization become defensive and react with increased resistance, inability to understand the benefits of a change, and protection of the status quo.

At times, opportunities occur that can be used effectively to change behavior or systems. Since a difficult but critical first step is accepting the need for change, a crisis provides a reason to get things moving quickly. A concrete reason to change is easier for most people to accept than the abstract promise that change is "needed to make things better." Caution should be exercised, however, to avoid manipulation that will undermine the leadership's credibility. In addition, it is foolish to believe that redrawing an organizational chart or rewriting a procedure will suffice to implement a change. Although management may declare a change effective on, say, a given date, generally staff need some time to learn and adjust to the new ways of doing things before the change is really in place.

In implementing integrative organizational forms, it often is helpful first to implement a form early on the continuum of organizational alternatives, such as direct contact (number 3 in Figure 2.1). This will be less intrusive, disruptive, and threatening to others in the organization, and will require somewhat more limited skills, than alternatives further along the continuum. As integrative managers develop and refine the skills needed for their new responsibilities and establish relationships and credibility across the organization, stronger integrative approaches can be implemented in an evolutionary way. Also, starting with only a few programs allows organizational learning that can be carried into additional programs that are started later. The possible exception to these patterns of evolution is the implementation of program organizations (numbers 8 and 9). These structures so drastically alter responsibilities, reporting relationships, control, and power distribution that a distinct break from the traditional structure based on functional departments is inevitable at some point during implementation. However, by first implementing an internal reorganization of departments into groupings that correspond to programs (number 5), the departments and their staff can be prepared for the final step of restructuring into a program organization.

Change as a Process

Many theorists have written about the change process itself, noting that a predictable series of events occurs when an individual and organization experience a change. Lewin (1958) observes that the change process occurs in three stages: unfreezing, changing, and refreezing. Much effort in organizational change is misdirected toward implementing new systems, when the people in the organization have not been "unfrozen" and are unprepared to give up the old. Until they see the need to give up the old, they will not consider the new. Where our experience and views diverge from Lewin's is in interpretation of "refreezing." Although new approaches and systems typically are institutionalized after they are introduced, we find that viewing this phenomenon as "refreezing" creates a static view of organizations. In practice, learning organizations, facing the types of changing environments found in health care, must be flexible and continually changing.

Recently, Perlman and Takacs (1990) have further developed the concept of the organizational change process. They compare it to Kübler-Ross's five stages of dealing with death and dying and add five additional stages needed to complete the transition to a new organizational state. The authors highlight the role that human emotions play in an organizational change process and encourage leaders to recognize and effectively deal with these emotions. For example, since organizational change requires people to give up their current methods of doing things, as well as symbols representative of their current practices and, often, social interactions with friends at work, they experience an important loss. This process of giving up the old is experienced as loss—a type of death—and, as in dealing with death, we must deal with the emotional process of letting go by experiencing (and allowing for) a period of depression.

The ten stages outlined by Perlman and Takacs include the following: equilibrium, denial, anger, bargaining, chaos, depression, resignation, openness, readiness, and reemergence. As Table 6.1 indicates, each phase has indicative characteristics or symptoms

Table 6.1. The Ten Stages of Organizational Change.

Phase	Characteristic/Symptoms	Action
1 Equilibrium	High energy level. State of emotional and intellectual balance. Sense of inner peace with personal and professional goals in sync.	Make employees aware of changes in the environment which will have impact on the status quo.
2 Denial	Energy is drained by the defense mechanism of rationalizing a denial of the reality of the change. Employees experience negative changes in physical health, emotional balance, logical thinking patterns, and normal behavior patterns.	Employ active listening skills; be empathetic, non-judgmental; use reflective listening techniques. Nurturing behavior, avoiding isolation, and offering stress management workshops also will help.
3. Anger	Energy is used to ward off and actively resist the change by blaming others. Frustration, anger, rage, envy, and resentment become visible.	Recognize the symptoms; legitimize employees' feelings and verbal expressions of anger, rage, envy, and resentment. Active listening, assertiveness, and problem-solving skills are needed by managers. Employees need to probe within for the source of their anger.
4. Bargaining	Energy is used in an attempt to eliminate the change. Talk is about "if only." Others try to solve the problem. "Bargains" are unrealistic and designed to compromise the change out of existence.	Search for real needs/problems and bring them into the open. Explore ways of achieving desired changes through conflict management skills and win-win negotiation skills.

5.	Chaos	Diffused energy, feelings of powerlessness, insecurity, disorientation. Loss of identity and direction. No sense of grounding or meaning. Breakdown of value system and belief. Defense mechanisms begin to lose usefulness and meaning.	Provide quiet time for reflection. Use listening skills. Employee and organization engage in inner search for identity and meaning. Offer approval for being in state of flux.
6.	Depression	No energy left to produce results. Former defense mechanisms no longer operable. Self-pity, remembering past, expressions of sorrow, feeling nothingness and emptiness.	Provide necessary information in a timely fashion. Allow sorrow and pain to be expressed openly. Be patient: take one step at a time as employees learn to let go.
7.	Resignation	Energy expended in passively accepting change. Lack of enthusiasm.	Expect employees to be accountable for their resistance, inaction, or actions. Allow them to move at their own pace.
8.	Openness	Renewed energy. Willingness to expend energy on what has been assigned to individual.	Patiently explain again, in detail, the desired change.
9.	Readiness	Willingness to expend energy in exploring new events. Reunification of intellect and emotions begins.	Assume a directive management style: assign tasks; monitor tasks and results so as to provide direction and guidelines.
10.	Reemergence	Rechanneled energy produces feelings of empowerment, and employees become more proactive. Rebirth of growth and commitment. Employees initiate projects and ideas. Career anxiety abates.	Ask and answer questions for mutual satisfaction. Redefine career, mission, and culture. Ensure mutual understanding of role and identity. Employees will take action based on own decisions.

Source: Perlman and Takacs, 1990, p. 34.

and associated interventions that a leader can employ to effectively take the individuals and the organization through the change process.

Developing and consistently using a standard approach to similar types of change in an organization will result in the creation of norms for change. By using similar interventions for similar phases of change, people in an organization can become familiar and comfortable with the change process, no matter what issue is being addressed. For example, open meetings might be held for interested parties to present the end result of the change and/or to gather ideas on how to address the change, or multidisciplinary workgroups might be developed as the norm for bringing about a change. Thus, people learn that if they will be dramatically affected by the change, they can expect to be a part of the group that plans and implements the change. These standard interventions will come to be expected and in themselves will be a reassuring constant in the change process. Also, others less experienced in managing a change process will have a standard to follow, which may help them to bring about the desired new state more effectively.

Tools for Managing Change

In designing a change process, the culture of an organization must be honestly assessed so that it can temper the strategy being developed. As we have noted, some organizational cultures do not tolerate change. In such organizations, the strategy for change not only has to deal with the specific activities that would support the desired change but also may have to have a primal strategy to counteract the organization's general tendency to resist all change. Possibly the culture itself must be changed to create conditions that more readily welcome and support change in general. In the culture that uses "because we have always done it that way" and "because it did not work the last time" as accepted reasons for not changing, the underlying beliefs and perspectives will have to be transformed. Incentives must be developed that reward individuals for changing their "tune" on maintaining the status quo.

Other organizational cultures may be conservative in nature, but when a need for change is clearly identified and understood, the organization wholeheartedly carries out the effort very effectively. In such an organization, the initial steps in the strategy must promote this clear analysis and identification of the definitive need to change.

All of the above discussion presumes that an organization has the luxury of time for assessing the need and bringing about a desired change. Sometimes, however, when change is called for, there is no time for slow adjustment; immediate change is necessary. In such a case, some of the same steps are taken, but they may be less explicit in nature and less obvious. When an organization is suddenly faced with a financial crisis, it most likely will be easy to illustrate the definitive need for a change. One solution would be for senior management to decide how a reduction in expenses or increase in revenue will be achieved; or the better alternative may be to determine a percentage of change that needs to be achieved and place the responsibility for realizing it on the middle managers. They will feel empowered by the challenge and will develop into an army of change agents.

Vision

Change requires a direction. This direction is set by a vision. The vision must be communicated effectively to those who need to participate in, experience, and commit to the change. A vision does not need to spell out the details of the eventual system, unless they are known for certain, but it must delineate some broad goals and some specific outcomes. The vision provides the guidance, direction, and motivation for change without stifling creativity or forcing people to behave in a particular manner.

Senge (1990) notes that the gap between a vision and current reality generates a creative tension that produces energy for organizational change. Vision cannot be created through analysis of past or current activities, no matter how sophisticated the analysis. Vision focuses on a future for an organization, whereas analysis focuses on the past. The limitations of analysis as contrasted with vision are illustrated by the analogy of someone driving a car with a blanket covering the windshield, looking in the rearview mirror.

Paradigms

Organizational vision is hard to create, largely because people have a set of beliefs and rules about how things in general, and their organization in particular, *should* function. These beliefs, or paradigms, regulate behavior and ways of thinking. They can be useful for providing order and regularity to behavior in organizations and in society in general. Through every activity that is consistent with an organization's or an individual's paradigm, that paradigm is reinforced. Organizations typically reward behavior that is consistent and discourage behavior that is inconsistent with their paradigms. Thus, paradigms not only are helpful for managing the routine operations but also are inherently restrictive to even thinking about other ways of doing things.

For example, until very recently the accepted paradigm of hospitals comprised a building with walls in which patients were treated. Activities of patient care outside of these walls were seen to be outside of the paradigm of a hospital. Even the term *hospital* had (and, for many, still has) the connotation of a building. Thus, hospital managers focused on inpatient care and considered home health care to be outside their scope of activities. How limiting and artificial this is from the perspective of what patients actually need! Nonetheless, many people responded negatively to suggestions that a hospital should be anything else. Since people who work within a particular paradigm typically are unaware of its limitations, it is people outside of hospitals who are more apt to question why hospitals should restrict themselves to inpatient activities. As this example shows, an organization's current paradigm does not provide the conditions for creating a vision, but instead restricts creativity.

Ackoff (1978) provides a true example that illustrates the different results that can be attained from different approaches. If you are asked to redesign the telephone system, and you start by determining the system's current problems, your efforts will be focused almost exclusively on remedying those problems. Although, with appropriate expertise, you may eliminate the problems, it is unlikely you will introduce any new features. However, if you begin by determining what features you would like to have in a telephone system and do not restrict yourself to your current definition of what a telephone system is (your current paradigm), you could well create something entirely new. This is just how the touch-tone telephone was developed. Its designers broke from their paradigm for how phones should work, which restricted "dialing a number" to actually turning a dial.

Breaking the limitations of a paradigm requires first recognizing that paradigms restrict creative thinking. Unusual approaches typically are required to remove those restrictions. For example, techniques such as brainstorming and thinking by analogy can be used. In brainstorming, criticism of ideas is not allowed. This encourages freewheeling thought and the generation of ideas that do not fit the current paradigm. Often such ideas are met with humor, as participants in the creative process are uneasy with violating their current paradigm. Thinking by analogy provides a way of getting away from the current issue by creatively dealing with one of its attributes and then bringing the solution back to the general issue.

We recently used both of these techniques to assist a hospital task force in developing an improved patient discharge system. The task force identified that ineffective patient transport delayed the discharge process. Hospital practice called for transporting all discharged patients to the front entrance in wheelchairs. Breaking from their current paradigm, some task force members noted that patients typically walk from the entrance to their cars, and questioned whether it was necessary to take all patients in wheelchairs. In continuing the creative process, members were asked to think about other places where large numbers of people were transported efficiently. Airports were mentioned. Imagining how people moved within airports, someone suggested that patients could be transported on people movers (moving sidewalks) or in vehicles like golf carts that could hold several patients. Some of these ideas appeared silly and "far out." Certainly they are nontraditional. But that is exactly the point: these ideas are creative and hold the potential for doing things in a substantially different way. Without getting beyond the limits of the organization's current paradigms, such approaches would not even be considered.

Some ideas generated through creative processes will not be feasible to implement. Some, however, hold the potential for a breakthrough. In beginning sessions on creative thinking we emphasize these points to participants:

- It is virtually impossible to make a current (and therefore, by definition, feasible) practice innovative.
- In contrast, it often is possible to make an innovative approach feasible.

Therefore, techniques of this type can be important tools for achieving the magnitude of change needed for many health care organizations.

Communication

Open and routine communication is the most important tool that we have to manage change effectively. From clearly explaining the desired change in terms that all individuals can understand, to actively listening to ideas on better goals and ways of achieving them, to hearing why the change is not desirable or seen as appropriate, to willingly answering questions and concerns about the change and its potential implications, communication sets the groundwork for an effective process.

Remember that with a change a new language may need to be employed. Among the communication goals may need to be the introduction and assimilation of new terms into the organization. In the health care industry, where there are clinical and nonclinical components, this may be an especially complex and important element of communication. As noted in Chapter One, when various terms have different meanings the difficulty and frustration in communicating about organizational change increase.

Most of the people in the organization will not understand management- and business-oriented terms. Using such terminology is almost equivalent to speaking a foreign language. We do not expect English-speaking people to understand French intuitively, nor do clinicians expect managers to understand all clinical terms without explanation. Why should we, as managers and change agents, expect people to intuitively understand the jargon of organizational change and development? Using such terms to introduce new, innovative organizational structures is usually not well received; it is seen as "jargon" and is divisive and ineffective.

It is extremely important to gauge just how foreign the new vocabulary will be to others and develop a strategy for introducing it into the language of the organization. Remember who the audience is and help the audience to relate to the concepts and terms in ways that are meaningful to it. In health care, the universal concern is patient care. Thus, when introducing a structural change to the clinical professionals of the organization, focus on the impact the change will have on patient care. Develop examples that the members of your audience can relate to and that will illustrate how the change will affect them.

Consistency in messages is critical, to limit confusion and misinterpretation. Test the meaning your intended communication conveys by asking others what it means to them. In major communication efforts, it is best to test the messages on a small group of individuals not yet privileged to early discussions before initiating widespread dissemination of information. It is risky to assume that the message you intend to send is exactly what others are hearing, especially when a change process is new to an organization and its concepts and terminology are foreign.

A major change process, such as the introduction of integrative approaches involving task forces or teams and empowerment of staff, should include a communications "campaign." It is important to repeat the objectives and methods of change to reinforce them and ensure they are heard. As in advertising, repetition is a key factor. In addition, different people seek information from different sources. Therefore, it is helpful to use multiple communication vehicles to communicate a clear and consistent message. This will increase the chances of communicating successfully to the whole organization and reinforce the awareness and importance of the change.

For example, a communications campaign was used by an institution undertaking a major construction project. Early in the process, the hospital recognized the emotional components of the project in terms of the impact the new building would have on individuals' jobs, workgroups, and routines, as well as the interim complications of water shutdowns, temporary moves, and constant noise. A campaign was developed to help overcome the emotional reactions to the project. In addition to the traditional media, such as the hospital newsletter and discussions at regular meetings, a good deal of effort went into new communication methods. Weekly open meetings followed by bulletins reported the status of the project. Individuals were encouraged to share concerns and ask questions about any aspect of the project. Meetings were scheduled with psychologists, so that people could talk about their emotional responses to the project. A resource team was developed and made accessible to all managers to support them in planning for temporary situations and for the final move to their new areas. Additionally, a project "hotline" was established. This gave people one number to call with questions, problems, and concerns, which then were dealt with expediently. Individuals who participated in the project expressed gratitude for the campaign because it promoted clear, consistent, two-way communication about the complex and sometimes overwhelming project. In the meanwhile, of course, it was "business as usual" at the institution.

Participation

In designing a campaign for change, it is critical to get people involved. Effective change is built on individuals' efforts. This fact cannot be avoided. Participation breeds commitment. It also is a source of mutual support and reinforcement for people dealing with ambiguity and stretching their skills to reach new goals. Take an inventory of people's resources in your institution, and possibly in the community, to know what help is available. Learn who the stakeholders are—in other words, who those individuals are who will be most affected by the change. Are they going to gain from the change, and thus be likely to support it? Or will they hinder the change because they expect it to bring them some kind of loss? Consider incorporating key stakeholders into the change process by making sure they have some influence over the process of change and its results. For example, can they lead an effort to look into a particular component of the change? Also, identify the people the stakeholders respect and are influenced by, and employ those people to help win the stakeholders over to the change.

Enlist "disciples" who can go out and communicate the purpose and benefits of the change and who can help promote acceptance of the change. Initially, senior managers should be the disciples, collectively supporting and consistently communicating the need for and the direction of the change. Lack of their support signals to others in the organization that the change will not really happen. Since the senior managers are seen by others as having influence and controlling important organizational resources, such as budget and personnel, their stand on the change is critical for its success.

Whereas senior management support is necessary, it is not sufficient. Disciples must be drawn from all levels of the organization. This is done most effectively by getting people involved in specific activities that give them a clearer understanding of the effort and eventually gain their commitment to the need for the change. In many cases, employees can communicate more effectively with their peers than the senior managers can. They may freely be asked, "What is really going on?" whereas that kind of question would never be raised in front of the senior management group. As was discussed extensively in Chapter Three, on integrative managers, disciples who have credibility and good relationships with their colleagues and other professionals, including physicians, can play a key role in influencing others—in this case, to support the change process.

It often is effective to enlist individuals who represent the major constituencies that will be affected or that need to be mobilized to bring about the change, and have peers introduce the concepts to peers. Nothing can take the place of a physician hearing from another physician why a particular issue must be supported by the medical staff.

Expect support to move through an organization outwardly in concentric circles. Early in the process, participation is limited to those committed to the change. As task forces and teams are developed, people who are unsure about the change but willing to participate join the initial supporters. The next ring of people generally are those who take a "wait and see" attitude. They can usually be brought into active participation only after the direction of change and the organizational commitment to it are clear, and some initial successes are achieved and reported. Finally, the outermost ring of people are the strong opposition. Some of them eventually will join the change process, and some will not.

Managing Meetings

A whole toolbox of methods exists for assessing the need for change and developing strategies for implementation, as well as gaining participation and commitment to change. Training people to run effective meetings is an important part of all change processes. Typically, much of the communication about the need for a change and how to effect it occurs in meetings. The effective management of groups and group dynamics can be critical in moving a process along, gaining commitment, and avoiding frustration. In structural alternatives that implement task forces or teams, group effectiveness is absolutely critical to success. Expectations in terms of ground rules for individuals and groups should be established and the ground rules reinforced. One effective way of doing this is by discussing at the end of a meeting how well a group worked together. Another is to list each person's expectations of others and to discuss these expectations, whether they seem to contribute to group effectiveness, and how to ensure commitment to meeting the expectations. For example, it is usually helpful to reaffirm that meetings will start at the scheduled time, and that people are expected to be there promptly. This often avoids a trial-and-error approach to determining how late it is acceptable for people to arrive.

In one setting, a group developed a list of its values and included an expectation that comments made on others' ideas should be constructive in nature and provide added value rather than rude critique. The group decided that anyone who violated this guideline would be required to put a dime into a "penalty jar," which was brought to all meetings. The jar was used symbolically to give negative feedback to someone violating the agreed upon values of a group. It also provided a nonthreatening way for someone who felt violated to so indicate. For example, participants found it much easier to say "That will cost a dime" than "I do not appreciate your sarcasm."

Off-Site Meetings and Retreats

Retreats are often used to initiate change processes. As discussed above, critical steps in any change process include developing recognition of the need for change, developing a strategy for the change process, and gaining commitment to the process. These take considerable time and can easily be interrupted by the normal distractions and emergencies of typical work activities. In addition, getting people to think about change requires shifting their focus from current activities. This is difficult to do in a hospital, where people's current responsibilities must take precedence. The shift of attention and the commitment to a new approach can definitely be reinforced through group dynamics, but often the time and attention needed to initiate such an effort cannot be found in routine staff or team meetings. Also, you may want to address a larger group than a team or staff meeting. In such a case, an off-site retreat is effective for getting individuals out of the work setting, and ensuring a major block of time is available for focusing on the change effort.

Total Quality Management

Total quality management (TQM) is a management approach and organizational change process directed at continuously improving quality. It holds great potential for health care quality improvement and is being used extensively by hospitals. Books have been written on TQM, a concept too complex for us to do justice if we tried to give a full description in these pages. However, it will be helpful to note the relationship between the organizational change efforts discussed in this chapter, pertaining to implementation of integrative organizational forms, and TQM.

Although several of the techniques that are incorporated in TQM are different from those discussed in this book, many are the same. TQM has the same philosophical basis as organization development. The two approaches are complementary and can be used together. TQM is value-driven by customer satisfaction, not only external customers but also internal customers in every segment of the delivery process. Central to TQM are collaboration across disciplines and empowerment of staff to identify problems and develop solutions. Integrative approaches discussed in earlier chapters seek the same objectives. The use of teams and task forces, the importance of participation and of managing group process effectively, the use of brainstorming and other group techniques, the need to orchestrate the change process, and the critical need for senior management's support of the process also are the same.

TQM also provides a set of terms and statistical methods that are concrete and often accepted more easily than the integrative approaches initially are. TQM's step-by-step approach provides a structure for finding and solving problems that can greatly assist integrative task forces and teams.

TQM does not explicitly address structural alternatives, however. By implementing an appropriate structural form, the objectives of TQM and the integration of disciplines can be better achieved. By changing its organizational structure, an institution's focus can be redirected more appropriately toward the flow of services to groups of patients. This will allow for implementing quality improvements more easily and provide an institutional basis for continuing new processes.

Other techniques presented in this book can also be used to augment TQM. For example, the concept of intermediate products is useful in the analysis of work flow, a key component of TQM. Caution should be taken, however, to avoid duplication of effort and overcomplication in the change process when both integrative organizational forms and TQM are implemented simultaneously. It is inappropriate, for example, to develop a steering committee for the integrative organizational changes and a separate quality steering council. One committee should provide oversight and guidance for all of the simultaneous change efforts. We have used the two approaches together and have found them to be mutually reinforcing.

Reinforcement of Change

A change process very likely will be a long series of events or accomplishments that over time, unless specifically identified, will not be readily felt or recognized. An effective change process is or-

chestrated and managed, with attention given to both the content
of the change and the process. Especially in organizations whose
culture is not supportive of change, it is important to build the
momentum of the change process and to reinforce the belief that the
change is not only possible but valued. To achieve this, it is important to reinforce and reward the people who are participating in the
change process. This will keep them motivated and committed to
the change and signal the desired behavior to the organization.

Often reinforcement can be achieved simply by identifying
accomplishments as they happen. Identifying a goal, achieving it,
and then receiving recognition for it can be a very motivating experience. Recognition can be provided through articles in the hospital newsletter, presentations at meetings, positive comments
about the efforts by the organization's leadership, in poster sessions
or displays in the cafeteria, through videotaped descriptions of the
change project and new vision, or through open discussions. When
time is taken to reflect on the change process, accomplishments can
often be identified. Small "wins" or achievements are better than
none at all and should be reinforced.

In beginning a change process and building its momentum,
it is important to choose issues that can be addressed successfully.
Every successful intervention will contribute to the belief throughout the organization that the change process is real and that change
is happening. Actual examples of change are much harder to deny
than are promises (or threats, to some) of change. In selecting issues
to address, it is often helpful to consider both the importance of the
potential change and the difficulty in achieving it. Often there are
issues that have moderate to high importance and are relatively easy
to achieve; these should be addressed first. Once the credibility of
the change process is established, efforts can be directed at more
difficult and important issues. If, however, no issues can be identified as both important and easy to achieve, it will be necessary to
begin with matters of lesser but still significant importance that are
relatively easy to achieve. It is essential to establish the credibility
and momentum of the change process before addressing issues that
are both important and difficult. Because important issues that are
difficult to achieve typically require development of support, move
at a slow pace, and do not attain results in the near term, they do

not initially contribute to momentum and support of the change process. Issues that are both unimportant and difficult to achieve should not be addressed. Others that are significant and achievable will continue to arise. In planning and orchestrating a change, in addition to determining the content of the change, an organization generally is well advised to follow the sequence we have suggested.

During the process of a change, there are times when it may feel as though nothing is going well and you are up against a mountain of resistance or conflict. It is good to remember that an organization undergoing a change process will experience "growing pains," and that times of conflict may be healthy signs of progress. These pains are sure to be felt when an organization challenges its most ingrained procedures or norms. It is important at such times to objectively assess where the organization is in the process. Do not reinforce the old ways of doing things. Try to refocus energies on making the change process move as it is intended to, reinforce the momentum by recognizing each step along the way, and proceed at a comfortable speed. When the magnitude of the change process seems overwhelming, it is often helpful to remember that "the way to eat an elephant is one bite at a time."

Conclusion

Recognizing the importance of the change process is as critical as knowing where the organization needs to go. We have used many analogies to explain the change process at an individual level. We are all well aware of the effects and stress associated with personal change for the individual. Organizations are made up of individuals, and the feelings and their significance for the organization are parallel to the feelings and significance experienced by the individual. In summary, we make the following points about the change process:

1. Organizational change is a physical, cultural, and emotional process; recognize and manage all of these aspects.
2. Although a change may have (and, it is hoped, does have) a positive objective, it may not initially appear as such to those who are affected.

3. A change process typically requires development of new skills and a new language.

4. Change is greatly affected by the culture of an organization; it often is necessary to change the culture to enable an organization to change other aspects of its functioning.

5. The paradigms that help to regulate the routines of an organization also stifle creativity and hinder change; recognize the power of paradigms and use creativity techniques to develop a vision that sets the direction for organizational changes.

6. It is nearly always impossible to change just one thing in an organization; identify the related implications of a change and prepare for them as well as possible.

7. Change can occur via evolution or revolution; although evolution is preferred because it allows time for learning and adjustment, revolution is sometimes required.

8. Change can progress at various speeds or not at all; avoid impulsive change as well as "paralysis by analysis," which can halt all change.

9. Change follows a process of fairly predictable stages; plan a change strategy that guides and assists people through these stages.

10. Ambiguity is inherent in a change process; recognize this as a fact rather than as a failure of the process.

11. Management tools do exist to plan, promote, and manage change effectively; use them.

12. Open and consistent communication is a key ingredient of an effective change process; manage communications and develop a communications campaign.

13. A change process will have growing pains; use them as events for reflection and learning and do not be discouraged.

14. Reinforce the desired changes; senior management's support for change is critical.

15. Frequently review accomplishments in the change process, to reinforce momentum and contribute to motivation.

Chapter Seven

Product Line Management: A Special Case of Integration

In practice, many integrative organizational innovations of the types discussed in this book have focused on product line management. In fact, in five of the six case studies presented in the chapters that follow, the hospital chief executives stated that they were implementing "product line management" or "service line management." In some situations, product line or service line management does contribute to organizational integration, with the product line or service line manager performing the role of integrative manager. However, in other situations integration is not an objective of the effort. Unfortunately, the terminology used to refer to "product line management" and "service line management," as well as to innovative organizational forms such as "matrix organizations," is inconsistent in both the literature and in practice. Therefore, it is difficult to compare various types of organizational alternatives.

Product line management has a negative connotation for many people in health care, especially clinicians. This is one reason why many have chosen to refer to their approach as "service line management." In addition, many organizations have been unsuccessful in implementing product lines or service lines. This has contributed to the view that product line management is a fad that has mostly passed. Given that there are several critical factors needed to implement an integrative structure, as discussed in Chapter Six, it is not surprising that there have been numerous failures. Also, when expectations are unclear, efforts to meet them tend to be seen as failures, and characteristics, advantages, and limitations of one variation of product line management have been confused with those of other variations.

Although product line management has a bad name in many quarters, it can provide many of the integrative advantages discussed in previous chapters. If it is poorly understood and inappropriately applied, it also can be trouble for a health care organization. This chapter will help to clarify the concept of product line management and relate it to the integrative organizational framework of the book. We begin with a review of the literature.

The Product Line Management Literature

In the search for better methods of organizing and managing, the health care industry has adapted practices used in other industries to its own purposes. Product line management is not new. The term and concept originated in 1928, when Procter & Gamble identified the need to centralize all data relative to individual products or "product lines" in order to optimize manufacturing operations and ultimately maximize profits. The first product to be given this focused approach was Lava soap (Dominguez, 1971; Anderson, 1985; Salter, 1986; A. J. Rice, 1987). "Procter & Gamble developed a system in which functional areas were coordinated to develop, produce, price, monitor, distribute, and promote this particular product" (A. J. Rice, 1987, p. 29). Dominguez (1971) refers to the need for operations to decentralize decision making and information in order to maximize profits. Manning (1987) credits General Electric and other Fortune 500 companies with utilizing product line management to spur growth of profits in the late 1960s and early 1970s. He estimates that 20 percent of the Fortune 500 companies have adopted a product line management approach.

The specific application of this industrial concept to health care has received both positive and negative critiques in the literature. Much has been said about the expected outcomes and benefits of product line management operation versus traditional approaches (Ruffner, 1986; Hoffman, 1986; MacStravic, 1986; Folger and Gee, 1987). There is general agreement that product line management is beneficial. These benefits fall into three categories:

- It promotes quick identification of the changes in the environment, patient demographics, case mix, and other information.
- It results in a better understanding of the impacts of changes in the environment and marketplace in addition to more accurate simulations of new strategies.
- It allows better allocation and control over resources and costs, quicker responses to changes in the environment, better implementation processes, and target marketing.

An additional benefit is product line management's consistency with financial and operational management requirements under the prospective payment system (MacStravic, 1986). In fact, several authors have argued that the tendency to move from the traditional hospital structure to more innovative approaches is a result of the dramatic changes in reimbursement (Fetter and Freeman, 1986; Charns, 1986; Manning, 1987). Hoffman (1986) views benefits in terms of continuity of care, distribution of limited resources to deserving and excellent services, and participation in decision making by professional care givers.

Several authors have noted differences in product line management approaches between health care and other industries. Manning (1987) argues that patients cannot be seen as the equivalent to a product; rather, they are consumers of services or products. From his perspective, the main impetus for using product line management in health care is the need to respond to DRGs and the prospective payment system. He questions, however, whether product lines for hospitals really exist and argues that the DRG system does not provide the necessary framework for defining a hospital's product lines.

Manning also states that the hospital industry is more constrained than other industries with respect to the ability to pick and choose the services they wish to provide. Manning states, "A basic core of services must be provided by all hospitals for licensure, ethical, operational, and image reasons" (p. 25). He argues that hospitals are limited in the "niches" they can carve for themselves, as the market will not support a low cost/low quality provider. Additionally, he argues that hospitals have limited investment capital due to a reduction in new hospital debt and equity financing caused by the uncertain environment and legislation.

Fottler and Repasky (1988) state that "the concept of aggregating patients into product lines may be viewed by physicians, administrators, and patients as too technocratic and indicative of an assembly line approach to hospital care that may adversely affect quality" (p. 16). The results of their survey also indicate that product line management, although viewed favorably by a majority of hospitals, is seen as most applicable to large, urban, for-profit hospitals and thus as less likely to be implemented by small, rural, not-for-profit hospitals. Communication and coordination concerns between top management and product line manager positions, resulting in a reluctance to delegate the required authority to successfully manage a product line, are also seen by Fottler and Repasky as issues affecting the implementation of a product line management approach.

Lowe (1987) points out differences between health care and other industries as well as the "hazards of the transition" from a traditional to a product line approach. The differences he notes are the overlaps in authority with physicians and their role, the power of third party payers and government, and the shrinking inpatient market. Hazards of transition were seen to be general chaos in terms of roles of product line managers; proliferation of overhead owing to discrete decision making; unproductive internal competition and strife, with neglect of essential services that are not yet part of product lines; emphasis on short-term profit versus long-term growth; and physician resistance.

The Confusion

A Touche Ross survey (1987) indicates that 48 percent of hospitals in the United States plan to implement product line management in some manner and that 75 percent of those hospitals with more than four hundred beds are currently utilizing product line management concepts. In a telephone survey conducted in California, Super (1987) found that 82 percent of hospitals have implemented, will implement, or are considering implementing product line management. Fottler and Repasky (1988) found in a survey conducted in Alabama, Florida, and Georgia that 58 percent of the respondents think it is likely that their hospital would adopt product line management. Yet, Nackel (1988) found that only 5 percent of hospitals have a product line or matrix organization. The specific definitions of the terms *product line management concepts, product line,* and *matrix organizations* used by those conducting and responding to these surveys, as well as differences in sample sizes and geographical areas of focus, help to explain the major differences in the results.

The wide differences in survey results illustrate two points. First, there is much variation and confusion in the use of product line management and related terms; the concept of product line management means different things to many different people. Second, there appears to be a great amount of interest, if not intrigue, concerning product line management and the advantages it offers for responding to the changing health care environment, and it is expected that a good percentage of the health care institutions in this country will eventually use some form of it.

Definitions of Product Line Management

Table 7.1 is a compilation of definitions of product line management and related terms used in the literature. The table also includes the various authors' assumptions of structure and authority requirements, and attributes of product line managers. The definitions differ in important ways. In some, *product line management* refers to a fully decentralized organization structure with separate and distinct business units as product lines. Each discrete business entity focuses all its energies on the research, planning, production, pricing, accounting, and promotion of a specific set of products (Nackel and Kues, 1986; MacStravic, 1986; Folger and Gee, 1987; Salter, 1986). This definition can also be equated to Patterson and

Table 7.1. Definitions and Terms for Product Line Management.

Author and Term	Definition	Structure and Authority	Product Line Manager and Attributes	Other
Patterson and Thompson (1987) market management model	"Emphasis is placed on market surveillance; overriding goal is to initially identify needs and opportunities and then to address them by developing innovations in health care delivery. The result is increased patient volume."	Marketing staff expanded, advisory role in pricing/cost containment issues, no formal authority, top management still maintains responsibility for responding, full-time market interface without tampering with traditional hierarchy.	Selling and marketing expertise, yet typically no professional sales experience; rather, administrative or nursing background.	Often represents first in a series of steps toward organization change.
Patterson and Thompson (1987) distribution management model	"Emphasis on managing channels of distribution—primarily physicians and organizations such as HMOs, PPOs. . . . The focus is on channel placement or the development of channels of access to the hospital. Its principal measure of success is increased utilization."	Department head designated as distribution manager, staff role with line responsibility for the department, responsible for recommending change to the appropriate people.	Business or planning skills, innovativeness, product line knowledge, computer literacy, ability to work with a variety of managers, and relationships with physicians.	
Patterson and Thompson (1987) strategic business unit management model	"Encompasses the most significant changes to traditional hospital hierarchy. . . . 4 to 8 distinct business lines organized around clinical, operational or market similarities without regard for whether the service is provided in hospital or nonhospital setting."	Traditional clinical hierarchy decentralized to general managers. "Top management's role is to provide overall institutional direction in business and clinical priorities, set financial policies and guidelines, and provide appropriate levels of staff and service department support for the product lines."	General manager responsible for "volume (utilization), profits (cost and prices), and strategy. Ongoing business planning, budgeting, and profitability management." Negotiates for services from departments not within business line (housekeeping, laboratories).	May be eventual outcome of the move toward product line management. "Some clinical roles may be centralized to ensure professional quality such as medical staff credentialing, and nursing quality assurance. However, their role would be one of staff support, not one of functional management control."

Table 7.1. Definitions and Terms for Product Line Management, Cont'd.

Author and Term	Definition	Structure and Authority	Product Line Manager and Attributes	Other
Salter (1986) product management	"The planning, direction, and control of all phases of the life cycle of products including the creation and discovery of ideas for new products, the screening of such ideas, the coordination of the work of research, etc."	Exact reporting relationships and responsibilities depend on needs of particular organization and specific product or product line being addressed. Requires "broad authorities throughout all phases of the organization."	"Charged with ensuring that cohesiveness is achieved throughout the organization." Total responsibility: research, development, finance, pricing, accounting, advertising, sales promotion. Marketing manager control over marketing research, production, sales promotion. Creative, flexible, and market oriented.	Benefits of approach can be gained without reorganizing total management structure.
MacStravic (1987, p. 36) product line planning	"Examining, monitoring, and forecasting activities of the hospital in terms of its products and product lines as a basis for making decisions about what services to offer, how, and to whom. The emphasis of most product line analysis has been on making strategic and operational decisions regarding which products to offer or where costs are to be controlled better." "Virtually all hospitals in competitive environments should be engaged in product line planning."	"Most product line planning includes the use of a technique called portfolio analysis. The purpose . . . is to determine which product lines are most deserving of investment versus which are risky or unpromising to expand or continue." "Requires that all hospital activities, revenues and expenditures be assigned to . . . product line categories."		

Source	Term	Definition	Notes
MacStravic (1986, p. 38)	product line marketing	"Product line marketing is responsible for recruiting and retaining the right numbers and mix of medical staff members. It is also charged with seeing to it that necessary patient volumes and patient mix objectives are met. . . . Product line marketing requires product line planning and benefits from product line management."	In contrast to product line planning, product line marketing can be introduced incrementally.
MacStravic (1986, p. 37)	product line management	"Requires organizing, directing, and controlling operations of the hospital in product and product line categories." "It introduces the possibility if not the necessity of conducting specific functions differently in distinct products or lines. Separate admitting and discharge procedures might be followed for obstetrics versus surgery versus medicine. If all functions of the hospital are to be operated in the same manner across all products and lines, there is no product line management. . . . Major emphasis . . . is cost control. Unlike traditional management efforts to control costs by controlling functional departments, . . . cost control works	

Table 7.1. Definitions and Terms for Product Line Management, Cont'd.

Author and Term	Definition	Structure and Authority	Product Line Manager and Attributes	Other
	primarily by influencing how physicians manage their patients . . . can be introduced incrementally by starting with separately managed programs such as the ER."			
Yano-Fong (1988, p. 27) product management = product line management	"Product line management is a planning and management system which coordinates and facilitates the services within a product line to provide comprehensive and cost-effective care to each patient."	Need to restructure is seen as potential disadvantage. "Most organizations change to a matrix structure." Nursing is potentially distributed "according to how it interfaced with the various product lines. . . . Nursing could either lose power in how it affects patient care or perhaps gain an important voice if within each product line, nursing had a significant impact on the product line."		Details pros and cons of using marketing strategies in health care: "Marketing plans enable hospitals to make optimal use of their resources . . . marketing strategies raise ethical concerns . . . because marketing is said to be the process by which people are convinced to buy products that they do not want or may not need."
Tucker and Burr (1988, p. 51) product line management	An approach that should be considered when determining the organizational design and process for executing the elements of the marketing mix.	"Under full development of this organizational design, a specific manager is assigned administrative responsibility for coordinating all attributes of an offering. . . . The model assumes the presence of a multifaceted executive at a relatively low level in the organization."	Production manager, financial manager, marketing manager: "Will the manager of a service have sufficiently broad skills to perform these effectively?"	"The benefits (speed, flexibility, and individualism of the service) must be balanced against the increased administrative costs of adding this layer of management to the traditional, functional organizational design."

Source			
Wodinsky, Egan, and Markel (1988, p. 222) product line management	"An organizational strategy and the management control system for addressing the programmatic scope of hospital operations."	"Product lines are superimposed over the existing functional organizational structure. . . . To provide leverage in motivating functional mangers, the product line manager should report at a relatively high level in the functional hierarchy, to the CEO, COO, or the senior VP, for example. . . . Product line managers have responsibility for reviewing and analyzing business units, introducing new, profitable lines, and guiding the marketing cycle. However, there are not many cases of product line managers with direct authority over the line's part of a functional department's operations."	"Product line managers are spark plugs, and cheerleaders for the line, generating enthusiasm and facilitating smooth operations through communication and problem resolution."	
Nackel and Kues (1986) product line management	"The organizational structure, management control systems, and delivery strategies for health care services structured around case types or major clinical services."	"Each product line should be a separate and distinct business unit within the hospital. . . . Each of these business units should be oriented as a profit/loss center. . . . Each business unit manager reports directly to the CEO or COO." Responsibilities include planning and delivery, defining costs, determining profitability, assisting in marketing efforts.	Who should manage? "The answer varies by type of business, teaching or nonteaching responsibilities, and individual people skills within the organization . . . Teaching hospitals would probably assign physicians as product line . . . managers. But community hospitals would be more likely to assign operations-oriented professionals to manage their product lines."	Utilizes Johns Hopkins Hospital as an example of how product line management can be delivered.

Thompson's (1987) "Strategic Business Unit model" and to position number 9 on the organizational continuum presented in Chapter Two.

In other definitions, *product line management* is a general term referring to a product- and market-oriented strategic focus that can be achieved by utilizing a number of different organization structures. Salter's (1986) definition allows for a range of applications, where product line management in its purest form aggregates specific services that can be developed, planned, marketed, and accounted for.

Product line management is also used to refer to a general product/market orientation being implemented in hospitals, which may be referred to as centers of excellence, service lines, macro segments, core business, business units, and management centers. This use of the term does not imply or require any particular organizational arrangements or structure to achieve the objectives (MacStravic, 1986; Salter, 1986; Wodinsky, Egan, and Markel, 1988).

Some hospitals have pursued the benefits of product line management but have purposely avoided the term. Often, avoidance of the term *product* stems from a desire to disassociate health care from negative connotations associated with manufacturing and business, or from physicians' negative responses to the term.

Whether the term *product line management* is used or not, many hospitals have introduced innovations that focus management attention on the outputs of the hospital. This is in contrast to their traditional focus on individual functional and professional inputs to the care process, in which no one department focuses on the whole system of care delivery or on any particular part of the environment associated with outputs. When the output focus is on an identifiable service, such as cardiology, it might be appropriately termed "product line" or "service line management." When the focus is on a segment of the market receiving an array of services, it might better be termed "market line" or "market segment management." Sometimes the two overlap. For example, the broadly defined set of pediatric services not only can be identified in terms of a medical specialty, and thus a service line, but also in terms of a specific market segment—children—and on that basis might be viewed as a market line.

A variety of definitions for a single term is not an uncommon phenomenon, as noted in Chapter One. For example, the term *matrix*, which is reported in several studies noted above, is not used consistently. Multiple meanings for a single term can virtually render the term meaningless, as it becomes necessary to ask each user how the term is defined and applied. The varying uses of the term *product line management* in health care have increased ambiguity everywhere it is employed.

Strategic Orientations

To reduce the confusion surrounding the concept of product line management and relate it to alternative organizational forms, it is helpful to consider why an organization is implementing a product line management approach. The framework presented here is based on the premise that an organization should be structured to facilitate achievement of its institutional goals. When evaluating product line management, it is necessary first to consider the organization's strategy and the goals and objectives that reflect that strategy. For example, will emphasis be placed on just a few areas of service or on a broad range? Will specific segments of the population be pursued? Will strategic advantage be pursued through emphasis on financial management, on quality and/or cost of service delivery, or on promotion of some or all of the organization's services? Once these questions are answered, it is easier to identify the individuals whose efforts are most critical to the success of the effort. Knowing strategy and objectives, one can use the framework as a guide to choosing an organization structure; determining the required skills, background, and influence of product line managers; and selecting the appropriate reward and information systems.

In our research on product line management and other innovative organizational arrangements, we have observed three distinct orientations underlying the organizational strategies. These strategic orientations we term *planning and marketing, budget and control,* and *service delivery.* These orientations may occur singly or in combination. For purposes of clarity, we will discuss each of the three approaches separately.

Planning and Marketing

The planning and marketing orientation places management's focus on segments of the population defined by services needed or other common characteristics. This gives an organization a specialized, consistent, continuous, in-depth concentration on each segment of its environment—a focus not traditionally available in hospitals. Central to the planning and marketing orientation is the development of business plans specific to each product line. Planning and marketing research are conducted to analyze market share, profitability, quality, needs, and opportunities. Packaging, promotion, and sales by product line may be found in this orientation. The primary purpose of these activities, using market segmentation techniques, is to increase revenues through consumer recognition of specific programs.

Characteristic of this method is analysis of the programmatic comprehensiveness of each product line. It often provides the organization a vehicle to access and prepare for future technological advances and other environmental changes. This orientation sometimes extends into actual implementation of the business plans developed, which will reflect one or both of the other strategic orientations. How the planning or the implementation is accomplished and how well it is done vary with the choice of organizational arrangements.

Some organizations have chosen to perform only the sales and promotion portion of this orientation. At an extreme, a telephone number may simply be established to coordinate the distribution of information to the public. Although a risky practice, an organization might promote one or more product lines without understanding their cost and revenue structures, without understanding the competition or how to achieve market potential, and without affecting service delivery. Raising false expectations concerning the availability of a program of care will not, in the long run, increase market share and could potentially reduce it.

Budget and Control

The purpose of the budget and control orientation is to determine the actual costs of providing specific types of care and comparing the costs with the associated revenues. This method has evolved out of the prospective payment system and the need to determine surpluses or shortfalls on diagnosis-related group reimbursements. Most institutions began to make these types of analyses immediately after the shift to DRG reimbursement. Even with this information, however, many organizations find it difficult to actually affect the costs of care, as there is no one person or department responsible for the entire continuum of care received by any patient. Additionally, it may be difficult to gain physicians' support in modifying practice patterns. Yet, the information on patterns and costs of care indicates that efforts can be directed at influencing physician practice and shifting organizational emphasis to different services.

Service Delivery

The service delivery orientation focuses on the effectiveness and efficiency of the delivery of care, usually by monitoring and modifying medical practice, and by coordinating functional inputs to the care process and advocating for the product line. This orientation addresses both the individual elements of the care process and their coordination, to ensure comprehensive, integrated care. Although the service delivery orientation occasionally is found in isolation, it is usually combined with and reached through an extension of the budget and control orientation or the planning and marketing orientation. In such cases, the other orientations have typically revealed that modifications to practice patterns and treatment protocols were necessary to increase the effectiveness and efficiency of care, and the organization shifts orientations to meet these needs.

Combinations of Orientations

In practice, the three orientations described here are often found together in various combinations. Planning and marketing, combined with service delivery, aims at providing progressive, state-of-the-art care while enhancing the quality and consumer convenience of the care process by product line. The combination may also promote its progressive and specialized care programs. Budget and control, combined with service delivery, reinforces the management of service delivery, and, depending on the types of information monitored, may focus on effectiveness, efficiency, or both. This combination places the primary focus internally in the organization, although an organization might come to adopt this orientation as a result of external pressures on revenues or the need to lower costs, or it might monitor patient satisfaction as a critical indicator of effectiveness.

When the external planning and marketing orientation is combined with the internal budget and control and service delivery orientations, a more balanced perspective can be attained, allowing the organization to be responsive to external opportunities.

Many organizations are unclear as to what objectives they seek through product line management. Thus, they are unable to make an informed decision about what organizational alternative will best contribute to the desired results. When the objectives of the product line effort are clear, organizational form, integrative product line managers, rewards, and information system can all be selected by applying the framework presented in the book. In the next section, the relationship between strategic orientations and organizational alternatives will be described.

Matching Organizational Arrangements
to Strategic Orientations

For each strategic orientation, only a few of the organizational alternatives presented in Chapter Two are suitable to promote effectiveness and efficiency. These alternatives are the ones that provide the most favorable balance among the specialty functional needs, the product line's needs, and the organizational cost to manage the structure.

The review of the product line management literature indicates an inconsistent use of terminology to refer to different organizational forms. Most confusing is that *product organization* is used in different parts of the literature to mean any of the parallel organizational forms or program organizational forms, as these terms were defined in Chapter Two. In discussing the match between organizational forms and strategic orientations, it is important that we be precise. Thus, we will refer to the organizational variations using the terminology presented in Chapter Two. The "programs" discussed in Chapter Two are "product lines" in the terminology of the product line management literature, and "program organizations" (numbers 8 and 9 on the organizational continuum, Figure 2.1) are "product organizations." "Integrative managers" are "product line managers," whose control over personnel and resources varies with organizational form, as discussed in Chapter Two.

Planning and Marketing

The strategic planning and marketing orientation can be achieved using variations of the parallel organization, from simple direct contact through teams (numbers 2 through 6, Figure 2.1). The parallel organizational form promotes integration and interdepartmental planning through the establishment of an integrative manager or a group having that specific responsibility. The choice of specific parallel organization variation depends on the level of integration desired.

The variations of the parallel structure are successively stronger organizational approaches to implementing planning and marketing. The limited strength of direct contact (numbers 2 and 3) is suitable for initial planning efforts or marketing where only a limited need for efforts of the functional departments exists. Where the marketing and planning function is organized to allocate responsibilities for specific product lines to different product line managers (number 3), direct contact can be implemented more consistently. Task forces (number 4) provide a forum for clinicians and managers from throughout the organization to interact, as they need to do to initiate a major new product effort. Teams (number 6), which require some internal reorganization of departments to dedicate staff to product lines (number 5), greatly enhance ongoing marketing and planning of a complex product line. This is most important, however, where a planning effort moves into implementation that requires the support and effort of other parts of the organization. If review and adjustment of plans is not desired, use of teams is an inappropriate organizational mechanism. In that situation, teams and dedication of staff both require greater organizational effort than is needed to achieve the limited outcomes desired.

The functional structure (number 1) is not effective for coordinating the perspectives or influencing the behavior of the functional departments to meet product line needs. Individuals with marketing and planning skills can be added to a functional organization (number 2), but unless these people use at least direct contact, they operate in isolation from the rest of the organization, thereby severely limiting their effectiveness. The two program organizational forms (numbers 8 and 9) and the matrix structure (number 7) provide more product focus and capability for integration of functions within each product than is needed for the planning and marketing orientation. The weaknesses of the product and matrix structures outweigh the benefits that can be effectively utilized when pursuing the planning and marketing orientation. In addition, the higher cost of managing a matrix structure makes it an inappropriate choice for this orientation.

The integrative product line manager in the direct contact structure would need the skills of a marketing specialist. This individual would have no direct authority or control over other parts of the organization and would report to senior managers responsible for product line management, possibly as part of a marketing department. Alternatively, depending on the size of the organization, a senior manager may don a second hat and provide those marketing skills to the development of a plan for a specific product line or lines.

As discussed in Chapter Three, in a task force or team approach, general management skills, interpersonal skills, and influence increase in importance because the product line manager must rely on these to gain the participation and support of clinicians and managers of functional departments. In addition, the product line manager serves as facilitator and staff of the task force or team. Medical skills, as well as other clinical and nonclinical specialty skills, can be provided by the involvement of people from other parts of the organization who are participating in the product line planning and marketing effort.

Budget and Control

The budget and control orientation also could be achieved via the direct contact (numbers 2 and 3), task force (number 4) or team (number 6) parallel structures. A financial analyst would be required to aggregate and analyze the necessary information and to present the analysis to the appropriately identified constituencies. No line authority or control over product line resources would be necessary. The arguments for choosing direct contact, task force, or team are similar to those made in reference to planning and marketing. Furthermore, the arguments against the use of the functional, matrix, and product structures are also similar to those made above.

Service Delivery

Of the three strategic orientations, service delivery requires the most integration, and has been the focus of the previous chapters. As noted in Chapter Two, integrative approaches are best addressed in most organizations with a team variation of the parallel structure. This can be achieved only partially by reorganizing functional departments into subunits corresponding to product lines (number 5). Although that variation will achieve a consistency of staff assigned to each different product line, it lacks the team structure as the formal vehicle for integration. The service delivery orientation can be achieved only to a limited extent with simple direct contact or task force variations of the parallel organization. Although they can facilitate patient transfers, serve as a focal point for coordination of service delivery, and provide a forum for addressing interdepartmental issues, these less robust parallel organization variations are not strong enough to serve as bases for on-going coordination, consistent advocacy for the product line in interaction with other parts of the organization, or management of service delivery.

As discussed in Chapter Three, in the team approach, the product line manager most likely would be a clinical manager, such as a nurse manager, who would assume product line responsibilities in addition to functional responsibilities. He or she typically would carry some personal influence from the functional line position. The balance of needed influence would have to be achieved through interpersonal skills and the credibility received from the organization's product line management objectives. Since a nurse manager typically performs a role in coordinating the delivery of care with the best interests of the patient and the institution at hand, expanding that role to follow patients throughout the continuum of care and to influence the delivery of services from the functional departments could favorably affect effectiveness and efficiency in the delivery of care. The product line role need not be restricted to nurse managers, however.

As also noted in Chapter Three, product line management could be carried out by a triad, representing nursing leadership, medical leadership, and administration. This triad may be led by one member of the group, or the authority may be divided among the three disciplines, depending on the issue at hand. Although such arrangements are not seen in other industries, the nature of the power distribution among medicine, nursing, and administration makes it necessary in some health care organizations. The triad makes for more cumbersome management than a single product line manager, but it is often the only viable option for implementing a product line approach.

Since the coordinating requirements for service delivery are even greater than those for planning and marketing and for budget and control, the functional structure (number 1) cannot meet them. A matrix structure (number 7) would be more than adequate, but in most settings the negative impact of the ambiguity and conflict inherent in a matrix outweigh its advantages over teams, and effectively functioning teams are sufficient. Similarly, the program organizational forms (numbers 8 and 9) would address the needs presented by the service delivery strategic orientation and would actually be easier to manage than a matrix, but for most health care organizations their weaknesses outweigh their strengths.

Combinations of Strategic Orientations

When service delivery and budget and control are combined, expectations of financial performance usually are established and greater changes in the traditional distribution of power are required. The need to alter the distribution of money and power inevitably leads to organizational conflict. Departments that have previously been powerful owing to their ability to generate large amounts of revenue may suddenly lose their clout and become servants to the product line masters. It is not unusual for product line managers to advocate for greater control and even the dissolution of departments such as nursing, which would result in a product organization form. Although from the perspective of the product line managers such action would facilitate management of their product lines, a broader organizational perspective reveals the inappropriateness of this action for most health care organizations, as discussed above.

When budget and control and/or planning and marketing are combined with service delivery, a more comprehensive and powerful product line management orientation is indicated. To achieve this end, at least a team parallel structure (number 6) is required. The more powerful matrix organization (number 7) provides an even greater organizational basis for the combination of strategic orientations and represents a balance between an organization's product line and functional needs. Because the matrix is the most complex organizational form, it should be used only by organizations that truly need the power of the matrix to manage product lines, and whose culture and conflict management skills are capable of sustaining a matrix.

At great cost to the functional perspective, a product organization (number 9) can be considered. (When all of the strategic orientations are combined, and product divisions are accountable for profits, they often are termed strategic business units [SBUs].) Although it is easier to manage than a matrix, a product organization's weaknesses typically outweigh its strengths for health care organizations. This is most critical in terms of recruiting, retaining, and maintaining the competence of the different professionals who are critical to a health care organization's long-term success. It should be adopted only by those few organizations whose size and reputation allow them to minimize the dysfunctional characteristics of the product organizational form. In practice, to address the limitations of the pure product organization, a modified product organization (number 8) typically is used.

When strategic orientations are combined, product line managers require more skills of a general manager, as discussed in Chapter Three. When all strategic orientations are combined, the greatest requirement is placed on product line managers' general management skills. If clinicians are chosen to provide a clinical perspective to product lines, extensive business management training is required. Product line managers should report high in the organization structure, typically to a vice president for product lines. In the matrix option, the product line managers should be placed in the organization at a level no lower than department manager, and as high as vice president of the product line. As in the service delivery orientation, the triad of physician, nurse manager, and administrator provides a politically acceptable alternative and results in the mix of the skills and influence required. In product organizations, direct line authority is provided over much of the required organization. Some interpersonal influence is required and a good deal of indirect control is provided through the control of resources.

Conclusion

As can be seen through the comparisons made in this chapter, product line management can be viewed as a special case of organizational innovation. Its various forms reflect differences in objectives, as reflected in strategic orientation and in degree of integration. The more integrative strategic orientations, which are those that include service delivery, require more organizational integrative focus.

The appropriate choice of organization form and integrative manager can be determined through application of the framework presented in the previous six chapters. Where product line management efforts have failed, the reasons often include the following:

1. lack of clarity as to the desired outcome of the effort, providing no guidance in choice of organizational arrangements
2. inappropriate choice of organization structure
3. inappropriate choice of integrative manager
4. lack of required organizational supports, in terms of distribution of influence, rewards, or information system

5.   lack of recognition of critical issues in managing the change
     process, and/or not allowing sufficient time for implementation

In conclusion, many beneficial changes in hospitals have been made under the rubric of product line management. It can be used effectively to develop innovative, integrative, organizational and managerial arrangements that provide a focus on patients and on delivery of integrated care and that reduce fragmentation. Unfortunately, in many instances, product line management is assigned the connotation of "assembly line medicine," which has limited its acceptance.

The terminology associated with product line management is not clearly defined, and its many variations have differing effects on an organization. We suggest, therefore, that managers first consider the organizational strategy and outcomes they want to achieve in implementing a product line approach. Second, avoid the term *product* and, using the framework presented here, determine the design of the organization structure and the choice of integrative managers. This will allow an effective analysis of the advantages and limitations of different integrative approaches prior to beginning implementation.

PART TWO

From the Field:

Lessons in Design

and Implementation

The following chapters present six detailed case studies of hospitals that implemented different forms of innovative, integrative organizational arrangements. They were chosen to represent a variety of objectives (strategic orientations), structural forms, characteristics of integrative managers, rewards, information systems, and approaches to implementation. The cases are presented in order of their degree of integration, beginning with a parallel structure utilizing direct contact in "Biscayne Hospital" and progressing to a modified program organization in "Hanna-Thorndike Hospital." In several cases, the initial integrative structure was altered, thereby placing it at a different position on the organizational continuum. "Waller Hospital" is presented as the final case because its primary focus is on the change process, rather than on structure. The organizational form for each case is noted in the following list:

Chapter	Case	Organizational Form
8	Biscayne Hospital	Parallel: direct contact
9	Philadelphia Hospital Medical Center	Task forces
10	Hilltop Health Services	Direct contact and teams
11	Bayview Medical Center	Teams (Triads)
12	Hanna-Thorndike Hospital	Program divisions
13	Waller Hospital	Task forces; focus on change process

For each case, a brief introduction is included to orient the reader to the major issues being presented. A similar form is used for the narration of all the cases, which includes general information about the institution, the purpose or strategic orientation of the innovation, and details on the organization design, selection of integrative managers, reward and information systems, and the change process. Since the institutions varied greatly in their experiences and accomplishments, the degree of focus on the different issues varies from case to case. Following each case, we provide an analysis to illustrate the concepts delineated in earlier chapters.

The names and locations of institutions described have been thoroughly disguised, but each contains the essentials of an actual situation, and the quotations are those of members of the actual organizations. As is the case in organizations, individuals do not always agree on how or how well various aspects of their organization are functioning. The reader should not be surprised by these disagreements.

The case studies present both positive and negative experiences. We hope that the case studies and their analyses will reinforce the use of the concepts in such a way that readers can learn from the experiences of their peers and support the development of effective and efficient organizational change in the future.

Chapter Eight

Are Two Hats
Better Than One?

Biscayne Hospital

The Biscayne Hospital case presents a community hospital with an initial strategic orientation of planning and marketing (see Chapter Seven), but with expectations that evolved to include budget and control and service delivery objectives. The case describes implementation of the integrative structure and selection of integrative managers, whom the hospital called product line managers. This organization structure was near position 3 on the organizational continuum (Figure 2.1). Clinical operations managers were given product line responsibilities in addition to their other responsibilities. They were given training in marketing and business planning, but little assistance or support in integrating their programs through the organization. They were expected to use direct contact to collaborate with physicians and others in developing and implementing services in their product lines.

The senior management group, especially the chief executive, became dissatisfied with the progress of the product line effort. The CEO terminated the effort, to the relief of all the product line managers. The case illustrates the limitations of direct contact, the complications inherent in having integrative managers serve in both integrative and operational roles, and the consequences of insufficient management information, as well as the effects of insufficient attention to rewards supporting the integrative effort. In addition, the case demonstrates the great difficulties in implementing organization change without the senior management group's having a clear and common vision for the organization. Further details concerning the concepts illustrated in the case are discussed in the analysis.

Biscayne Hospital

David Davis, president and chief executive officer of Biscayne Hospital, was not pleased with the accomplishments of the hospital's product line management effort. In implementing product line management, he had hoped to increase the hospital's market share and revenues and to improve its operational effectiveness. Mr. Davis had seen no evidence, in the one year since the product line managers had been trained, that these objectives were being achieved. Competition among area hospitals was intense, and although the hospital did not lose market share, it also did not gain the volume that Mr. Davis had expected. In addition, relationships with medical staff were becoming more difficult, and changes in reimbursement were diminishing the hospital's financial performance. It was now more important than ever to ensure the most effective use of the facility's resources and ultimately to enhance market share. Based on the lack of success with product line management, Mr. Davis terminated the effort, but he was not sure exactly what other changes to make to replace the product line approach.

The Setting

Biscayne Hospital was a 277-bed private, not-for-profit community hospital located in Miami, Florida. Miami had a large elderly population and a large Hispanic population. Competition among hospitals in the city was intense, and each hospital looked for ways to uniquely distinguish itself. Biscayne Hospital enjoyed a modern physical plant, designed to provide a pleasant milieu for its patients.

Biscayne Hospital was known as a doctors' hospital, having been founded in 1955 by a group of doctors dissatisfied with another hospital in the city. Although Biscayne Hospital had no medical school affiliation, in several specialties its medical staff were acknowledged leaders in the region and had large practices serving patients referred by primary physicians. The medical staff were quite vocal about their needs and those of their patients, but no physicians were members of the hospital's senior management group.

Mr. Davis had been the chief executive at Biscayne for eight years, and had been hired because of his expertise in financial management. In 1983 the hospital faced severe financial difficulties, resulting primarily from debt incurred during an aggressive building program in the 1970s and from a declining census. The board of directors had considered mergers with other institutions, as well as outright closure of the hospital. Instead, Mr. Davis was recruited to address the hospital's severe financial situation. He was given extensive latitude by the board. Within three years of his arrival at Biscayne, Mr. Davis had successfully reversed the hospital's trend of increasing financial deficits, and the hospital had shown modest financial surpluses each year since 1986. During that time, Mr. Davis also terminated many long-term senior managers and recruited an aggressive new senior management team.

The Organization

Figure 8.1 represents the organization of Biscayne Hospital. Mr. Davis served as president and chief executive officer. Senior managers with line responsibility reporting to Mr. Davis included the chief operating officer (COO), the vice president of finance, and the vice president of medical affairs. Staff positions that reported directly to the CEO included the heads of planning and marketing, human resources, risk management/quality assurance, and development. Harold Gordon, who played a major role in the hospital's product line management effort, was vice president of planning and market-

Figure 8.1. Biscayne Hospital.

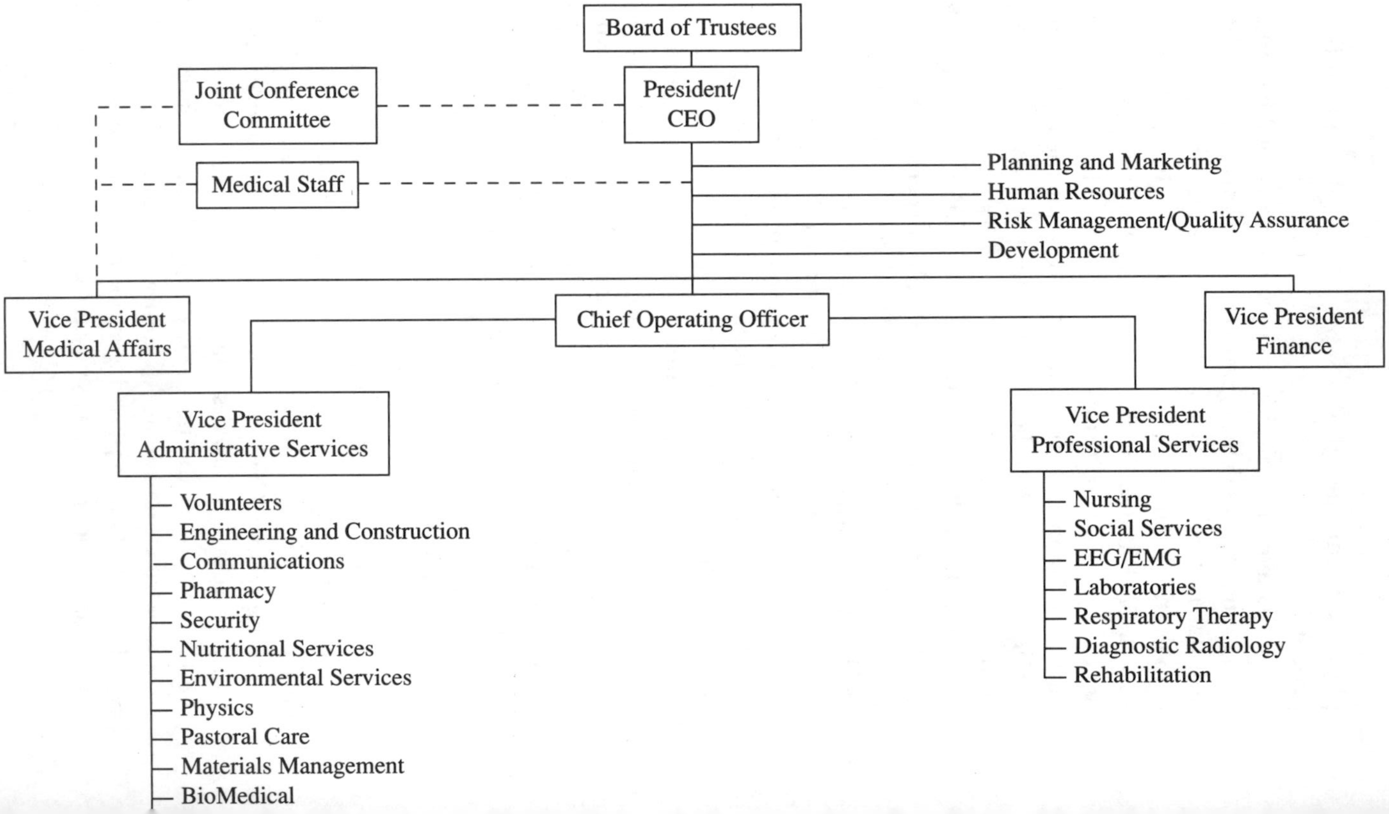

Board of Trustees

President/CEO

Joint Conference Committee

Medical Staff

Planning and Marketing
Human Resources
Risk Management/Quality Assurance
Development

Vice President Finance

Vice President Professional Services

Nursing
Social Services
EEG/EMG
Laboratories
Respiratory Therapy
Diagnostic Radiology
Rehabilitation

Chief Operating Officer

Vice President Medical Affairs

Vice President Administrative Services

Volunteers
Engineering and Construction
Communications
Pharmacy
Security
Nutritional Services
Environmental Services
Physics
Pastoral Care
Materials Management
BioMedical

ing. He also was responsible for public relations, sales, and physician services. Robert Fischer was vice president of human resources, and Lee Taylor was vice president of finance.

The COO position was held by Julie Coleman, who had come to Biscayne in 1986. Reporting directly to the COO were the vice president of professional services, Carol Anderson, R.N., and the vice president of administrative services, Cal Stone. All department managers reported either through the vice president of professional services or the vice president of administrative services.

The senior management group was led by Mr. Davis and included Mr. Gordon, Mr. Fischer, Ms. Coleman, Mr. Stone, Ms. Anderson, and Ms. Taylor.

The Culture

The culture of Biscayne Hospital reflected the personality of its dynamic CEO. It was an aggressive organization where it was "not possible to work too hard." Mr. Davis communicated high performance expectations for his management team and did not want to hear excuses for why something was not accomplished. He also promoted risk taking, and no idea was too outrageous to entertain. However, it was not uncommon to see a lot of effort devoted to a project and then see it brought to a sudden halt.

Managers believed that the typical Biscayne Hospital employee had a higher productivity level than counterparts at other hospitals, but was also paid better. Many senior managers stressed that Biscayne Hospital attracted strong-willed, hardworking individuals who were willing to pull together to continue to move the hospital in a positive and progressive direction. The managers wanted to be a part of this hard-driving organization and were willing to make compromises needed to achieve desired results. Many of the senior managers had come to Biscayne specifically for the opportunity to work with Mr. Davis.

The institution's senior managment focused on the financial, strategic, and synergistic implications of any given project versus the organizational and cultural implications. Outcome was emphasized over process. One product line manager expressed that the administration at Biscayne Hospital expected a lot from its managers as compared with other hospitals, and there was a clear focus on profitability. He elaborated, "We live and die by the numbers here." Additionally, the time frames for measuring success at Biscayne Hospital were typically very short; a year often was considered a long time.

One senior manager indicated that Biscayne Hospital had a "show and tell" relationship with its medical staff. With respect to organizational issues, such as product line management, the senior management team would not consult with the physicians prior to implementation. However, the senior management team felt its relationship with the medical staff was a good one.

Initiating Product Line Management

In 1986 Harold Gordon was hired as a new vice president. Mr. Gordon had extensive management and consulting experience in marketing and planning. Upon his arrival, Mr. Gordon initiated intensive market research. The research focused on the institution's specific competition, and segmented the market according to the way people look for services rather than by how hospitals prescribe to provide them. Mr. Gordon explained that "a broad definition of competition was used, to include any provider or product seen by a potential customer as an alternative."

The senior management group began to see the benefits of and need for providing marketing and management attention to the categories of services that resulted from the market research. Although the senior managers did not adopt the terminology initially, Mr. Gordon and his staff conducted research on product line management activities around the country. Ultimately, a commitment was made to develop a structure that would allow the institution to be proactive in preparing for the future. In addition to Mr. Gordon, the CEO, the chief financial officer (CFO), and COO were also driving forces behind the effort.

Three major objectives of the product line management effort were identified:

- increase market share
- increase revenues
- improve operational effectiveness

Additional organizational needs were identified for resolution by the innovative management approach:

- a two-way communication system for physicians that would provide a focal point to direct all correspondence
- an orientation that would facilitate the quick development of coordinated business plans
- an organization structure that would cut across functional lines and strengthen the bonds between departments

The next step in implementation was defining specific product lines. This was found to be a difficult process, and consumed a considerable amount of the planning and marketing staff's time. The staff analyzed discharge data according to various groupings of DRGs, but were unable to determine any grouping that corresponded satisfactorily to medical specialties or to segments of the population previously identified through market analysis. Mr. Davis, who was frustrated by the amount of time consumed by this process, stated, "It does not matter how you define your product lines. It is whatever makes sense for our organization." Mr. Davis was also very surprised with the greater-than-expected number of "turf issues" that emerged between departments and within the senior management group during the definition process. Eight product lines, not defined strictly by DRG, were finally identified by the planning and marketing group:

- cardiology services
- gerontology services
- orthopedic and rehabilitation services
- oncology services
- women's health services
- emergency services/trauma center
- general medical services
- general surgical services

The Selection of Product Line Managers

Following the definition of the product lines, product line managers were selected in September 1987. The new positions were not posted by Human Resources. Instead, senior management selected product line managers from among the hospital's managers and supervisors. There was no opportunity for interested managers or staff from either inside or outside the hospital to apply for the new positions. The positions also were not formally graded by Human Resources, and job descriptions were only broadly defined. Several of the managers initially chosen decided not to participate.

Most of the people who accepted product line management positions were middle managers from nursing or other clinical departments within the hospital. They had a range of clinical backgrounds. Six of the eight were registered nurses, and most were managers of patient care areas. The product line managers retained their departmental responsibilities, thus assuming two hats. The following list presents the product line managers' functional responsibilities and corresponding product lines.

Product Line	Functional Responsibility
Cardiology services	Director, Cardiology Department
Gerontology services	Director, Adult Day Care Center
Orthopedic and rehabilitation services	Director, Rehabilitation Medicine
Oncology services	Director of Radiation Therapy
Women's health services	Head Nurse, Labor & Delivery Unit
Emergency services/trauma center	Head Nurse, Emergency/ Trauma Services
General medical services	Clinical Coordinator, Nursing
General surgical services	Director, Operating Room

Product Line Structure

Responsibility for supervision of the product line managers was divided between the COO, Ms. Coleman, and the vice president of professional services, Ms. Anderson. The six product line managers whose functional responsibilities were in nursing were assigned to Ms. Anderson for their product line responsibilities; the two others were assigned to Ms. Coleman for their product line responsibilities. There was discussion within the senior management group of eventually having all the product line managers report exclusively to the COO, but this step was not taken. However, although they did not report to him, Mr. Gordon provided a good deal of support to the group. The new organization was presented at several board and medical staff leadership meetings. The structure was seen by the medical staff as a management issue and not a clinical one.

The product line managers had no formal authority beyond that which they held in their functional management roles. No additional personnel were assigned to them. They did not have control over any additional funds. Marketing money was appropriated for use by the product line managers, but its use had to be approved by senior management. Other departments were not reorganized to specifically provide service and support to the product lines. For example, individual social workers did not provide services exclusively to patients of any single product line. The product line managers could contact HMOs but could not negotiate with them, since the hospital contracted with HMOs on a hospitalwide basis.

In most cases, the managers had no formal business backgrounds and depended on the training and support they received from the department of planning and marketing. To augment their business skills, Mr. Gordon conducted a seven-week training program for the new product line managers. The program included a general orientation to marketing, data sources, data analysis, alternative organization structures, including matrix organizations, and a review of the development of business plans. This process occurred from November 1987 through early January 1988. (See Table 8.1 for a timetable of product line management activities.)

In January 1988, the product line managers were charged by the senior management team with developing their individual business plans. The business plans were to be developed by the end of

Table 8.1. Product Line Management Timetable.

Harold Gordon hired	1986
Preliminary planning completed	September 1987
Orientation of managers	November 1987–January 1988
Business plan development	January–March 1988
Business plan presentations	April–May 1988
First six-month review	November 1988
Scheduled second six-month review	May 1989

March 1988 and presented to the senior management group during April and May of 1988. Product line managers were responsible for addressing questions raised by senior management. Follow-up meetings, in which each product line manager provided status reports to the senior management group, were scheduled to occur every two to three months.

The product line managers were given guidance in developing business plans by Mr. Gordon, who recommended that they include general information about the product lines and their specific products, as well as detailed information and analysis of the market and marketing strategies. A financial analysis was to be conducted, including cash flow and break-even analysis. The management structure and organization of the product lines were to be described and were to identify key individuals, labor force considerations, and legal issues. An implementation plan was to be outlined, indicating potential problems and an estimated time line with benchmarks and milestones. The product line managers were encouraged to use budgets, exhibits, and articles to support their plans. After the first business plan presentations, the product line managers were asked to complete strategic action plans outlining three-month work plans for each of the components of the business plan.

Rewards

All managers were evaluated using a management-by-objectives system, which had been implemented shortly after Mr. Davis's arrival at Biscayne. Each year, managers met with their superiors to set goals for the coming year and to determine measures for those goals.

Goals typically focused on implementing new processes, cost savings and efficiencies, and personal professional development. Salary increases were based largely on the achievement of these goals.

Both goal setting and performance appraisal activities were scheduled to occur annually during the month of November, although typically the schedule was not strictly followed. Product line goals had not been incorporated into the management-by-objectives process. Therefore, product line managers' evaluations with Ms. Coleman or Ms. Anderson were formally based only on achievement of departmental goals.

Information System

To conduct the analyses and develop the business plans, the product line managers required information detailing Biscayne Hospital's performance and that of its competitors. Mr. Gordon and the planning and marketing staff oriented the managers to the various internal and external sources of data. Sources of external data included state agencies and the Florida Hospital Association. The product line managers were also given consulting reports comparing volumes of different procedures among geographical sections of the state.

The internal information system, similar to that in most hospitals, basically tracked clinical and financial data on inpatients. It was necessary to reaggregate these data to meet the product line managers' needs. The director of finance and the product line managers agreed that it was a struggle to get the information needed to support the product line management effort. By late 1987, the Finance Department had installed a new cost accounting system, but a history of costs identified by product line had yet to be developed. The product line managers did receive monthly department performance reports, revenue reports, and census reports for those departments that were relevant to their product lines. The Planning and Marketing Department also was used as a resource for information.

Further Evolution of Product Line Management

In November 1988, six months after the first presentations were made, the senior management group had grown dissatisfied with the process, as the group did not see the results that it had initially anticipated. At that point, the senior management team made no changes, but agreed to evaluate the progress of the product line management effort in six months.

At about the same time (late 1988), the product line managers brought their concerns to the senior management team. A number of the product line managers argued that the loosely defined structure and lack of authority limited their effectiveness. The product line managers sensed a difference of opinion within the senior management group about the concept and structure of product line management. Ann Waters, product line manager of cardiology services, expressed views typical of the product line manager group: "The organization did not understand the concept. There was a difference of opinion at the senior management level, the middle managers felt threatened, and the staff were unsure where they fit. Additionally, I consistently felt that my first priority and responsibility was the operation of my department."

When they addressed the issue to the senior management team, the product line managers expected that the administration would act on their recommendation and provide them with more authority. However, it eventually became apparent that the level of authority was not going to be changed.

Although no formal evaluation of product line management had been conducted, in May 1989 Mr. Davis decided that it was time to step in to correct the situation. He reflected:

> In retrospect, I see we should have acted sooner. We had clear objectives for the effort, but in implementation we missed our target by a mile. The senior managers never totally agreed on the reporting relationships or implementation plan. We wanted the product line managers to run with the ball, but we didn't agree on the game plan. In addition, the medical staff, Carol Anderson, and many other clinicians and some administrators objected to the term "product." They could not relate it to the service orientation of the hospital. This had serious consequences for success.

Product line managers and senior managers both felt it was difficult for the product line managers to fulfill both departmental and product line responsibilities. Senior managers expressed the following opinions:

Ms. Anderson: It was difficult to keep the product line managers motivated to develop the strategic outlook while meeting the other needs of running the institution. It was confusing for the senior managers, too. For example, how could I tell nurse managers to ignore the operational needs of their areas? I found it very stressful, and so did they.

Ms. Coleman: Changing from an operational focus to a strategic focus was difficult. As long as product line managers had operational responsibilities—and that was our design—the effort was not going to work.

Mr. Fischer: Product line responsibilities were a lot of work for people who were already very busy. The fuzzy definition made it even more time consuming. As a result, from the start it was going to be tough to succeed.

Joseph Martin, product line manager of oncology services and director of radiation therapy, offered views typical of the product line managers:

> I went as far as I could go. I had to tease others to get involved, and this was very time consuming. It was the old story of having responsibility but not authority. Without the authority, we might as well disband. I had no control over what happened on the oncology unit. I did not get the census reports and could not influence staffing levels.

Outcomes of the Product Line Management Effort

The product line managers did feel a sense of accomplishment. They had developed new programs as a response to the needs of their market segments. Some had successfully developed influential relationships with managers over whom they had no direct authority and with medical staff, and they had substantially increased their business skills.

Mr. Martin: I felt that the process worked fairly well at getting different parts of the organization to work together despite the turf issues that we encountered.

Maria Cruz, product line manager of women's health services: Product line management could combine patient advocacy and business. I bridged the gap between clinical services and the Planning and Marketing Department by ensuring appropriate and accurate advertising. I also perceived my role to be that of expediting other people's priorities.

I had to regain my credibility with the operational managers, who felt somewhat displaced organizationally, and to make the operational managers feel as though they were contributing something of value. There certainly has been some organizational pain and discomfort. I recommended that the senior management communicate the rationale of the selection process to middle management.

Mr. Martin: I saw my role as making people in the hospital aware of the programs available, to increase and improve communication, and to develop a strong relationship between the medical staff and administration. I saw myself as the mediator between physicians and administration. The physicians and administration do not often get to hear each other's ideas. Product line management provided a medium for this communication to occur.

Ms. Waters: I certainly developed a clearer understanding of what my department's particular needs were.

Concern was expressed for the time frames that were established and the conflicts the product line managers encountered in trying to achieve their goals.

Ms. Cruz: I became inundated with my strategic action plans, and there were differences of opinion on what was a reasonable amount of time to get things done. Additionally, some of the programmatic objectives conflicted with the increased revenue objective. For example, the shortened maternity stay program, which reduces length of stay via an educational program, could actually contribute to a reduction in revenue.

Mr. Martin: The physicians in my department were uncomfortable with the product line management push. They were happy with the share of the market that they held and were concerned that the new program ideas would jeopardize the trusting relationships that they had developed with referring physicians. Product line management should not always be directed toward financial issues. It should focus on service delivery issues.

Several product line managers mentioned the management-by-objectives system and the intrinsic rewards of the position.

Marcia Harding, product line manager of general medical services: The hospital never acknowledged the importance of product line goals. Our product line business plans were presented to senior management, but the management-by-objectives system never reflected these goals. It was schizophrenic for us.

Ms. Cruz: There were intrinsic rewards received from the position, as I had the ability to develop programs in response to community needs and to see the projects through from beginning to end. The product line management title was seen as a disincentive, however, from the perspective of the physicians. Many believed that hospitals did not manage products and saw the effort as just another administrative structure. A second disincentive was the visibility of the position and the need to openly deal with controversy. This effort became wearisome, and I began to question, "Am I really in charge?"

In the spring of 1989, David Davis saw the need to end the organization's product line management effort, as it had not achieved the desired goals of increasing market share, revenue, and operational effectiveness. He called the product line managers individually into his office and told them that the product line management effort, as they knew it, was being halted. Most of the product line managers felt relief.

Still believing in the benefits of a product line management approach, Mr. Davis wondered how to redesign the method Biscayne Hospital would use to manage its services.

Case Analysis

Biscayne Hospital exemplifies both the advantages and the limitations of the direct contact parallel organization form. Compared to other organization structures, direct contact is inherently limited in its potential for integrating across hospital departments. When implemented effectively, however, direct contact provides a management focus on individual programs. Clinical managers usually have firsthand information and experience to use to lead the development of clinically relevant programs and effective relationships with medical staff.

Only limited benefits of direct contact were attained at Biscayne Hospital. Other organizational factors prevented the product line managers from overcoming the conflicts and ambiguity inherent in their dual roles and developing influence throughout the hospital. Senior managers did not agree on how the product line arrangements would function, nor did they provide clear support to the product line managers. The hospital's information system provided little assistance to the product line managers, and the lack of rewards for integrative efforts indicated to the product line managers and others in the hospital that product line management was not a priority. In addition, Biscayne Hospital's approach to organizational change itself limited the potential for success.

Strategy and Structure

Biscayne Hospital's approach to product line management was driven by a planning and marketing orientation, with the possible addition of the other two strategic orientations, budget and control and service delivery (see Chapter Seven). This approach appears appropriate for Biscayne Hospital, given its history, competition, and strengths in the market, especially if service delivery and budget and control receive increased emphasis as the process evolves.

There is serious doubt, however, about the clarity of the hospital's objectives and its commitment to them. For the most part, the organization acted as if the objectives were limited to planning and marketing. A key driver of the effort was Hal Gordon, the vice president of planning and marketing. Training efforts were focused on market analysis and planning, product line managers received their greatest support from Mr. Gordon, and they were directly charged only to develop business plans. Yet the senior managers stated the objectives more broadly: increase market share, increase revenues, and improve operational effectiveness. To some degree, the senior managers' dissatisfaction with the results of product line management may have stemmed from lack of clarity about what they really wanted to achieve. In fact, some new programs were planned and some relationships with medical staff were developed. Direct contact is appropriate for budget and control and for planning and marketing, but it is insufficient to achieve integrated service delivery, as noted in Chapters Two and Seven. Thus, it was unrealistic to expect that the product line managers could improve operational effectiveness using direct contact. At a minimum, this required use of task forces and, preferably, teams.

To achieve the limited objectives, it was appropriate that product line managers were given integrative responsibilities without formal authority or control over resources. Contrary to the need expressed by many of the product line managers and contrary to traditional management paradigms, control and formal authority are neither required nor inherent in the parallel organization forms. The success of direct contact depends directly on the ability of integrative managers to persuade other managers and clinicians that their collaboration will achieve improved outcomes for patients, for the clinicians themselves, and for the hospital. With success in achieving these outcomes, the integrative managers' influence will grow. But integrative managers need senior management's support and assistance, as well as rewards and information for their integrative program efforts, especially during the initial phases of implementation of direct contact. These elements were lacking at Biscayne Hospital and, together with ineffective management of the change process and its short time frame, they the precluded the success of product line management.

The use of direct contact was further compromised by the fact that the product line managers had significant other responsibilities in addition to their product lines. Although they received support from the Planning and Marketing Department, the product line managers were clinicians first, clinical managers second, and integrative managers third. The product line effort was more abstract than clinical management; the product line managers were not completely comfortable with their new responsibilities, and they had not fully developed their business skills. Thus, when problems developed in their areas of functional responsibility, they were inclined to address those issues rather than work on the less tangible and less immediate business plans. This was reinforced by the formal rewards. As Ann Waters stated, "I consistently felt that my first priority and responsibility was the operation of my department."

Structurally, the reporting relationships of the product line managers also did not facilitate integrative management. As noted in the case, responsibility for the product line managers was divided between the COO, Ms. Coleman, and the vice president for professional services, Ms. Anderson. Reporting to the same person for both functional and product line responsibilities did not assist in distinguishing between the dual responsibilities. The case also notes that the drivers of the process were Mr. Gordon, the CEO, the CFO, and the COO. While Ms. Anderson was not a driver of the system, she was the individual to whom six of the product line managers were accountable. This must have created some ambiguity for the product line managers and left a void in the support they needed.

A more appropriate structure would be one in which the product line managers were accountable to individuals other than those in their functional line of authority. Additionally, the senior managers responsible for the integrative efforts should be people who are clear advocates of the new approach. If Biscayne Hospital wished to emphasize a planning and marketing approach, then it would be appropriate for the product line managers to report to Mr. Gordon. If service delivery were to be given greater emphasis, then reporting to the COO would be appropriate, as long as the COO was a clear advocate for the effort and the objectives of the effort were clear.

Selection of Integrative Managers

The product line managers were clinical managers who were known entities at Biscayne Hospital. Recognizing the managers' deficiencies in business skills, the Planning and Marketing Department provided an orientation over a three-month period. The time frame for accomplishments was aggressive, especially with the product line managers' having dual responsibilities. With a longer time frame, clarity of objectives, and support from senior management, the initial product line managers quite likely could have developed their integrative skills and built on their established clinical relationships.

Although the dual roles of the product line managers were cited as a problem at Biscayne Hospital, the arrangement of dual roles can work. Its advantages are that it allows an organization to build on the competence and influence of known members of the organization and to implement the new arrangement without the cost of new full-time positions. At Biscayne Hospital, however, the inherent confusion about dual roles was compounded by the lack of clarity among senior management and by the short time frames and the need to develop new skills, which overloaded the product line managers. To relieve the product line managers, it would have been prudent to assign some of their departmental responsibilities to functional subordinates. In addition to providing time for the product line managers to devote to their integrative responsibilities, this would have provided a vehicle to develop new management talent.

Alternatively, Biscayne Hospital could have selected senior managers to assume integrative program responsibilities in addition to their traditional responsibilities. This has both advantages and disadvantages. Since senior managers do have greater formal authority and influence than other managers, giving them integrative responsibilities indicates the importance of the effort to the rest of the organization and assists in initial steps in implementing integrative programs, as discussed in Chapters Three and Six. However, this arrangement does not empower lower levels in the organization. Without formation of task forces, it does not facilitate the input of ideas from those in the organization closest to the delivery of care. Finally, it does not contribute to the development of future managers. In Chapter Thirteen, the Waller Memorial Hospital case demonstrates how clinical department managers can lead task forces with direct involvement of senior managers, thereby achieving all of these advantages.

Rewards

Biscayne Hospital did not alter its formal evaluation and reward system to reinforce integrative efforts. Product line managers were rewarded for departmental efforts exclusively. This was especially problematic in that many of the product line managers were having difficulty shifting the focus of their efforts. Feedback and praise of the product line managers' efforts were limited, largely because their supervisor was unclear and uncommitted. Furthermore, when they requested clarification from the senior management group in late 1988, they did not get it. Some medical staff were negative about the effort, and there is no indication of strong support. Accomplishments of product line managers were limited, and thus they did not experience many intrinsic rewards from the job. Together with the lack of solid support from senior management, the lack of specific rewards left an ambiguous picture of the commitment to the effort.

Information System

Market data appropriate for the competitive analysis of the product lines were available to the product line managers. However, internal information on costs and operations was lacking. Thus, unless it limited its product line efforts to a marketing and external planning orientation, Biscayne Hospital lacked needed information. The dearth of information impaired not only the effectiveness of decision making but also the integrative managers' credibility and influence. Although the information system was being enhanced, it was not available during the short time given to the implementation of product line management.

The Change Process

The changes expected at Biscayne Hospital amounted to too much, too soon, without adequate time given to building the strong foundation of relationships and system supports needed for the new positions and new way of functioning. The initial effort was completely reliant on the Planning and Marketing Department and on the individual product line managers, who were given mixed signals about expectations of the effort. No organizational vision was created, and, in fact, little was communicated to the product line managers or the organization in general about the purpose or goals of the effort.

Several quotes in the case indicate that Biscayne Hospital was not process oriented. The risk-taking aspect of the culture, "where no idea was too outrageous," could have provided encouragement for organizational innovations. However, since developing an integrative organization requires altering relationships and expectations, it requires attention to process issues. Without managing the change process itself, its success was in doubt from the start.

One of the most serious problems at Biscayne Hospital was senior management's lack of support for the change. Given the culture of the organization and the fact that many members of the senior management team came to Biscayne to work with Mr. Davis, it could be expected that senior managers would want to innovate. However, there is no evidence that they had a shared vision for a new way of working as an integrative organization. By shifting power in the organization, the product line management effort could have been threatening to the senior managers. The new approach also was a sharp contrast to the old paradigm at Biscayne Hospital, in which the managers had been held individually accountable for results. Furthermore, the effort was highly reliant on the vice president of professional services, who was unclear about its purpose. For example, she noted, "How could I tell nurse managers to ignore the operational needs of their areas? I found it very stressful." Doubts, questions, and inconsistencies among senior managers in an organization soon and easily become known throughout the rest of the organization. Developing a consistent understanding and commitment among senior managers was a critical missing element in the hospital's change process.

Mr. Davis succeeded in improving the hospital's financial performance, but it is not clear that he had a vision for its future. At best, a shared vision was held by Mr. Davis, Mr. Gordon, and a few other senior managers. They did not appear to have a plan for implementation, and they did not communicate a vision to medical staff or others. Although the hospital was founded by doctors, relationships between medical staff and administration became fragmented, and under Mr. Davis there was a "show and tell" relationship with its medical staff. This conflicted with one of the key elements of the integrative effort and was a major obstacle to overcome. The product line managers themselves had the responsibility to communicate with the medical staff. The product line management terminology was not well received, as it had manufacturing connotations. Furthermore, middle managers were not well advised on the purpose of the effort. No broad communication about the effort, clarification of responsibilities of functional and product line managers, or incentives for cooperating with the product line effort were apparent.

The product line managers also faced some inherent conflicts that they could not resolve. The expectation of increased market share was not a goal that was shared by the medical staff who had to play a major role in providing referrals to achieve it. The senior managers felt that they could lead and the medical staff would follow. Given their somewhat distant relationship with the medical staff, Biscayne Hospital's managers needed first to establish the new effort as something that would benefit the medical staff. They had to earn credibility for the effort. This is best done by presenting issues in terms understandable to the clinicians and by achieving small but important initial successes on which more difficult efforts can be built. By leaving the medical staff out of any significant activities, management missed an important opportunity to benefit from the physicians' ideas and to gain commitment to any product line plans.

Outcomes

There was evidence of some achievements resulting from the effort. Where it was initiated, the medical staff did get more involved in planning and problem solving. Product line managers learned new business skills and developed a better understanding of their market. In addition, some integration was achieved, leading to new program development.

The successes of the product line effort can be attributed to the integrative approach, the personal efforts of the product line managers, and the efforts of the planning and marketing staff. Biscayne Hospital attained some of the outcomes that could be expected from the use of direct contact, and these are most evident in new program planning. The effort was self-limiting because senior management neither understood nor supported it, and the reward and information systems were inadequate. The change process itself was a significant factor limiting Biscayne Hospital's success.

Better guidance in the decisions about organizational arrangements and change could have prevented the major stress and cost of the Biscayne Hospital change effort while yielding more favorable outcomes. Much could have been gained just by implementing task forces and eventually evolving to teams. However, these would have required both time and senior management's support. Without clear objectives, any road (or no road) will lead them there.

Chapter Nine

Involving Physicians
and Trustees:

Philadelphia Hospital
Medical Center

This case presents a teaching hospital's experience with an integrative effort, which it termed "product line," and which was focused primarily on strategic planning and marketing. Although the intent of the effort was sound and responsible, the management of the process and the long time required to reach conclusions resulted in disappointed participants and, ultimately, results that were less than satisfactory.

Philadelphia Hospital Medical Center (PHMC) was closely affiliated with a medical school, and the school's agenda was highly intertwined with that of the hospital. The medical school department chairmen were the hospital chiefs of service, and they had considerable influence over hospital activities and direction. They also were very traditional in their thinking about management, strategic planning, and marketing. Thus, a significant challenge was to gain the chiefs' input and commitment to planning and setting new directions for PHMC.

Historically, the hospital had been organized purely functionally (number 1 on the organizational continuum shown in Figure 2.1). With the introduction of the product line strategic planning process, the hospital established large multidisciplinary task forces, led by "planners" (number 4 on the continuum), and including physicians, board members, and administrators.

Much can be learned from this case in terms of managing change, the strengths and limitations of a task force approach, and decisions as to leadership, size, and constituency of the task forces. The case is a classic example of the consequences of neglecting to get people who have a significant stake in the outcomes of decisions involved early enough in the process. It also provides an opportunity to consider how the design of the effort relates to the involvement of physicians and trustees and the time frame for accomplishments.

Philadelphia Hospital Medical Center

In July 1989, S. Jonathan Winthrop, M.D., president of Philadelphia Hospital Medical Center, was wondering what steps to take to continue the hospital's product line management efforts. Dr. Winthrop had just received a notice of resignation from Daniel Appleton, vice president of external affairs, who had accepted the position as chief executive officer at another hospital. As Dr. Winthrop thought through the implications of Mr. Appleton's resignation and how best to deal with them, he reflected on the hospital's strategic planning process and the achievement of the efforts that Mr. Appleton had led. In the previous two and a half years, the hospital had expended a great deal of effort on the product line oriented strategic planning process. Dr. Winthrop wondered whether it had met its objectives, what other benefits had been attained, and if it had been a wise investment of time and energy. He ultimately wondered what steps to take next.

The Setting

Philadelphia Hospital Medical Center was a 380-bed teaching facility in Philadelphia, Pennsylvania, offering a full range of services except for obstetrics and pediatrics. The hospital was the principal tertiary teaching site for the University of Philadelphia's School of Medicine. The medical school also depended on Philadelphia Municipal Hospital (PMH), adjacent to PHMC, to round out a full complement of services, including obstetrics and pediatrics, for the teaching program. PHMC also had several collaborative programs with PMH.

The hospital's central-city location, bordering several ethnically mixed and economically poor neighborhoods, had not proven to be conducive to the development of a strong outpatient service. This ultimately increased PHMC's dependence on its inpatient program. Additionally, lacking pediatrics and obstetrical services, PHMC did not have a good primary care base from which to draw. Therefore, it was very dependent upon its referring physicians. Its competition included several well-respected facilities: Albert Einstein Medical Center, Hahnemann University Hospital, Hospital of the Medical College of Pennsylvania, Hospital of the University of Pennsylvania, Temple University Hospital, and Thomas Jefferson University Hospital.

The Organization

PHMC had a traditional functional organization structure in which each department represented a professional or nonprofessional function. No organization chart had been developed at PHMC, a reflection of Dr. Winthrop's belief that an organization did not benefit from having its structure charted. The major reporting relationships were well known, however. In addition to legal counsel and the development officer, six vice presidents reported to Dr. Winthrop. Joyce Parker, executive vice president of operations and assistant to the president, was responsible for all operations other than nursing and planning. Reporting to Ms. Parker were two vice presidents of clinical operations, Madeline Cox and Kevin Carter.

Ms. Cox was administratively responsible for clinical nutrition, dermatology, diagnostic vascular laboratory, epidemiology, nuclear medicine, nutrition services, psychiatry, pulmonary laboratory, radiation medicine, radiation physics, radiology, respiratory therapy, social work, and the laser center.

Mr. Carter was administratively responsible for admissions/reservations, cardiology, home health services, laboratory medicine, materials management, neurology, occupational health, pathology, rehabilitation medicine, and the Felscher Institute. (Founded in 1922 through a major endowment, the Felscher Institute of Clinical Research and Preventive Medicine funded many of the efforts of the department of medicine.)

Also reporting to Ms. Parker were the assistant vice president for patient affairs and the administrator for plant operations. Ms. Parker retained the direct responsibility for anesthesiology, gynecology, institutional review board, tumor registry, management information center, medical records, oral surgery, quality assurance, the continence center, the Delaware Valley Male Reproductive Center, and the Henderson Eye Center.

Other people reporting to Dr. Winthrop were the vice president of human resources, Tina Keller; the senior vice president of nursing, Lee Lund, R.N., M.S.N.; the vice president for external affairs, Daniel Appleton; the senior vice president for finance, Norman Carroll; and the vice president for marketing communications and public affairs, Edward Houseman.

The medical staff structure reflected groupings by medical specialties. The attending physicians were medical school faculty, who in addition to clinical responsibilities had educational and research responsibilities at the medical school. Full-time paid chiefs of service were responsible for representing their departments administratively to both the hospital and the medical school.

The Environment

Prior to the prospective payment system and the development of alternative delivery systems, such as health maintenance organizations, individual physicians were able to work rather independently of one another. The advent of HMOs portended dramatic change in the teaching hospital referral system. HMO patients belonged to captive medical groups, and it was difficult if not impossible for programs and individual specialists to attract patients directly. One chief of service noted: "Previously, it was the hospital's responsibility to keep its stars happy. Now survival is dependent on the ability of the star to support the hospital. Working together [with other physicians to provide a continuum of care] previously had not been essential for excellence; now it is impossible for the individual physicians or specialties to work alone. Generally, physicians in a teaching institution can be compared to the bears in Yellowstone Park; they want to put their mark as high on the tree as they can."

One hospital manager stated: "The chiefs have recognized that they have to move from their individual intellectual units to economic units, but this move is not an easy one. The chiefs are a seasoned group of physicians and are actually facing a culture shock in having to face the environmental changes."

As a teaching hospital, PHMC had multiple and often conflicting missions. The very nature of a teaching setting led to conflicts between the medical school and the hospital and between the medical staff and the hospital in terms of mission, goals, objectives, and strategies. To maintain a well-rounded teaching program, the hospital needed to sustain a fairly full complement of high-quality programs. This, in itself, conflicted with the economic need to distribute the scarce resources of the hospital responsibly. One physician noted that it could probably be justified as a wise business decision if PHMC were to devote all of its resources to becoming the leading cardiothoracic center. If it made this move, however, PHMC would lose its medical center status.

Unfortunately, all of these commitments did not lead to consistent directions for the medical school and the hospital. The conflicts among service delivery, teaching, and research also were found within hospital departments. One medical chief indicated that the mission of the chiefs of service was beyond that of the hospital; this was why they seemed to work independently from the hospital. Another chief described the teaching hospital to be a truly "different animal" because of the limited administrative influence, the implications of teaching, the layers of bureaucracy, and the transient nature of researchers. Many people within and outside the hospital commented that, owing to the organization structure and relationship with medical schools, the administration of a teaching hospital, as compared to a community hospital, typically has less control over the direction of the institution.

To be effective, Dr. Winthrop needed the support of the chiefs of the major clinical departments. The chief of medicine, Paul Martin, M.D., who was extremely influential owing to his control over the wealthy Felscher Institute, had maintained continuous leadership since 1972. This had provided the basis for cooperation between the hospital administration and the department of medicine and its subspecialties. The other major department, surgery, had had two chiefs in the previous two years and, consequently, had been difficult to work with. Recently, the highly respected and influential chief of neurosurgery, Sam Edwards, M.D., had been appointed to the position of chief of surgery.

Organizational Strategy

Prior to Dr. Winthrop's assuming the presidency, PHMC had pursued a strategy of creating a network of strong community hospitals, striving to be the leader in such multi-institutional arrangements in the region. Its success was limited, however. The former chief executive often entered into such arrangements without medical staff support. In addition, few community hospitals saw the concept as desirable. PHMC, however, did enter into some contractual arrangements encouraging regionalization. One acquisition, an alcohol addiction center, filed for bankruptcy one month after its purchase.

The previous president saw no place for new buildings in the PHMC corporate plan. His vision was for PHMC to be the low-cost teaching hospital in the city. When Dr. Winthrop became president, he did not pursue such outside arrangements, but rather focused his energies on the much-needed building program. Thus, in February 1983, shortly over one year after Dr. Winthrop became president, an application was filed with the state for a replacement facility. In November 1985, ground was broken for the Center Pavilion, and in February 1989, patients were admitted to the new inpatient facility. The pavilion was promoted as a symbol of the "new" PHMC: a symbol of the renewed commitment to provide "the services that patients, families and visitors want from hospitals," and to support "talented, compassionate, and professional staff in the provision of the most advanced medical care in a manner and setting that makes patients and visitors welcome guests."

Previous Planning Processes

PHMC had previously seen the need for strategic planning. Efforts in the 1970s were said to have had no power base and thus were rather ineffective. Dr. Winthrop indicated that the hospital's planning process had always been "whatever the school was doing." In 1983, Sheila Lang, then vice president of external affairs, initiated a new planning process. Dr. Winthrop commented:

> The process was an obsession of Sheila's, and it was her determination that moved the process along as far as it did. The Lang process was very data driven. The focus of the process was to define the hospital's mission and relevant goals, objectives, and strategies, utilizing a broad market assessment.
>
> The process did not intimately involve the chiefs [of service]. Thus, it was clear that the medical staff did not buy into the results of the process. Surgery was in a state of flux due to the turnover in chiefs, and Dr. Martin, chief of medicine, did not enthusiastically support the effort, although he did not block it.

Dr. Winthrop felt that the planning process made people in the institution think about things outside the hospital's own four walls. He stated: "It helped PHMC see the need to replace the chief of surgery at the time. However, after the final planning document was compiled, it was never referred to again."

In August 1986, Ms. Lang left the hospital to assume a position as chief executive officer of a community hospital, and in 1987 Mr. Appleton was hired.

Product Line Strategic Planning Process

In 1986, there was general agreement among senior managers, medical staff leadership, and hospital trustees that PHMC needed a new and improved planning process. As the competitive and reimbursement issues were not expected to improve, and admissions and length of stay were declining, the administration, key physicians, and board members recognized that a decision needed to be made concerning the strategic direction that the institution would need to take to survive.

Mr. Appleton, a consultant for a local firm specializing in strategic planning and product line management, was recruited in January 1987 to fill the recently vacated vice president of external affairs position. Mr. Appleton convinced Dr. Winthrop to try a strategic planning process to identify a limited number of areas in which to concentrate resources; this would structure decision making needed to respond to the environment. The process was presented as a management decision-making process, based on internal ideas rather than pure data, and as a process in support of the physicians. It was a fast-track approach to planning that was expected to be completed within three to four months.

Dr. Winthrop needed to sell Mr. Appleton's idea to key board members and medical staff leaders. He proposed that the new process would provide a commitment of money and other resources to those groups of physicians who could work together to propose clinical program expansion or enhancement. The physicians would be required to estimate and commit to a projected number of new admissions that would result from the new or expanded programs. These projected volumes would be utilized in determining the financial feasibility of the programs.

The money was to come from reserves from operations. Typically, the hospital's annual new program budget was approximately $1 million. It was anticipated that approximately $4 million would be devoted to new and expanded programs resulting from the strategic planning process.

Initially, Mr. Appleton spent two months interviewing approximately one hundred people within the medical center about their perspectives on a future direction for PHMC. Dr. Winthrop believed it was critical to bring together administrative, trustee, and medical staff leadership to get the constituencies' ownership and commitment for the planning process. Therefore, in May 1987, he scheduled a retreat.

Retreat. In May 1987, Mr. Appleton conducted a retreat for over eighty trustees, administrators, and medical staff leaders. From Mr.

Appleton's perspective, the purpose of the retreat was to present evidence of the shrinking market share and to develop a structure that would facilitate a strategic planning process designed to increase, rather than just maintain, the hospital's market share.

To help present the competitive picture and identify areas of potential opportunity for developing leadership positions, the participants at the retreat were presented a list ranking PHMC, compared with its competitors, by services. PHMC ranked itself first for cardiology and geriatrics.

The physicians present at the retreat solicited a verbal commitment from Dr. Winthrop that money would indeed be allocated to programs that could prove their viability. Thus, Dr. Winthrop publicly stated that funds would be provided to expand or initiate viable services.

At the conclusion of the retreat, the group had suggested five strategic categories in which institutional energies should be focused:

- inpatient admissions
- graduate medical education
- multihospital arrangements
- diversification
- managed care

People held conflicting perspectives with respect to the success of the retreat. Some described it as merely a forum for airing ill will, while others felt it was a huge success in achieving the objective of gaining wide involvement.

Inpatient Census Task Force. The inpatient admissions effort was brought to life with the establishment of the inpatient census task force. The task force was chaired by Gisele Rouselle, an investment banker and member of the board of trustees. The inpatient census task force had a total membership of twenty-two people that included board members, medical staff leaders, and administration. The task force was charged with identifying the first steps that should be taken to increase inpatient census. Its tasks included identification of the first areas for market emphasis across clinical disciplines as well as identification of physician department opportunities for increasing census.

The inpatient census task force, armed with the cliché "We cannot be all things to all people," agreed that the hospital must focus its energies and resources on a small number of areas. Initially, the task force identified twelve market segments. To reduce the number of areas, the task force developed the following criteria, which the areas of focus and their markets would be required to meet:

- a growing market on an inpatient basis
- a large target population
- a service that is already strong at PHMC
- existence of general commitment by PHMC to the service

Dr. Winthrop had anticipated that from the twelve market areas, the inpatient census task force would identify three areas of emphasis where the strategic planning monies could be concentrated to expand current programs. However, according to Dr. Winthrop, the task force did a poor job of discriminating and thus identified seven areas of emphasis. He admitted, "I was disappointed when seven areas were identified, as together they represented virtually everything that PHMC did. The physicians were not skilled at trading off. The concept of singling out a few programs to emphasize is not consistent with the medical school requirement for a full complement of high-quality services."

Market Planning Teams. The inpatient census task force established market planning teams for each of the seven focus areas, which began to be referred to as "product lines." They included cardiovascular diseases, geriatrics, trauma/critical care, neurosciences, cancer, respiratory/pulmonary, and musculoskeletal. The market planning teams were asked to explain how their product lines related to the criteria established by the inpatient census task force and to develop a marketing plan for each product line. The marketing plan was not expected to indicate promotional activities, but to identify the resources required to expand or implement programs that would result in increased admissions. The teams collected, developed, and analyzed data on admissions, revenues, and estimated expenses for each specific program within their product lines.

In choosing the chairs of the market planning teams, Dr. Winthrop selected respected clinicians who would fairly represent all of the different services and functions that constituted each product line. Other members of the teams were either John Breugger, Ph.D., or Victoria Hitch, of the external affairs division; one of the three senior vice presidents of operations, Joyce Parker, executive vice president of operations, or Kevin Carter or Madeline Cox, vice presidents of clinical operations; representative nurse managers; attending physicians who were full-time medical school faculty; and referring physicians. Dr. Breugger and Ms. Hitch served as facilitators and staff to their teams. (See Exhibit 9.1 at end of chapter for market planning team membership.) The market planning teams' activities took the external affairs staff away from some of their regular responsibilities, which some managers felt resulted in a cost to the institution.

The musculoskeletal group dropped out despite the fact that it had a "star" physician leading the effort. This group saw the future of its line in the outpatient arena, and therefore its growth activities were not consistent with the efforts of the inpatient census task force. The respiratory/pulmonary group disbanded because the physicians involved were primarily research oriented, and they felt that the AIDS market would come regardless of the programming and marketing efforts. All of the remaining areas of focus except cancer met the criteria developed by the inpatient census task force. However, even though the institution did not have a well-developed inpatient cancer program, senior managers felt that the market was there and that the hospital should be better organized programmatically to meet the needs of cancer patients. Therefore, they allowed cancer product planning to continue as part of the strategic planning effort.

The programmatic focus required physicians from different specialties to work together. For example, the cardiovascular line required that both cardiac surgeons and cardiologists come together as a united front to justify, develop, and implement programs. Following is a sample of the aggregation of services in the five product lines that were initially pursued:

- *Cardiovascular Services:* cardiology, cardiac surgery, vascular surgery
- *Geriatrics:* geriatrics, psychiatry, rehabilitation medicine, general medicine, neurology
- *Neurosciences:* neurology, neurosurgery, rehabilitation medicine, psychiatry
- *Trauma/Critical Care:* emergency services, general surgery, neurosurgery, critical care
- *Cancer:* surgical oncology, medical oncology, radiation medicine

The market planning teams developed their reports and provided them to Dr. Winthrop. In reviewing the reports, the operational and financial managers who had not been members of the marketing planning teams expressed concern with the estimated costs of operations. Dr. Winthrop then asked these managers to become involved with the process. They repeated the financial analysis for each program, utilizing more conservative expense and revenue estimates and financial indicators. Formal internal rates of return and return on equity tests were conducted, using a very conservative hurdle rate. Based on the second financial analysis, Dr. Winthrop decided which programs would be given the resources identified as necessary for implementation. Excluding the cancer group, which had lacked a medical leader, all market planning teams received approval to enter into the implementation phase of the project.

Implementation Planning Teams. The market planning teams were converted to implementation planning teams. Ms. Parker advocated for the operations managers to take a leadership role in the implementation process. Mr. Appleton, however, argued to have the external affairs staff continue in their facilitation role. The final decision was to have the teams continue to be chaired by the medical chiefs but be facilitated by Ms. Parker, Mr. Carter, or Ms. Cox (executive vice president of operations and vice presidents of clinical operations). The external affairs staff members were no longer formally involved; they continued to participate when their previous experience with program development was helpful and needed. More than one source indicated that the operational managers privately relied on the external affairs staff because of the physician relations that the external affairs staff had cultivated.

The implementation planning teams provided their final reports to Dr. Winthrop in June 1989. Two of the four reports met their original target date, one was late by one month, and the other was late by two months. The final approval for the implementation of the new programs had, in some cases, occurred more than two years after the process had been originated. Although different people had different ideas concerning the impact of the process itself, by the end of 1989 management had decided, independently of the process, to spend $2.5 million of the $4 million allocated to the four areas.

Each of the four product lines had pieces of its program implemented. Proceeding independently, timed with the opening of the new building, promotional campaigns for "heart care, care for older people, neurosciences, and trauma and critical care" were developed; advertisements were placed in the *Philadelphia Inquirer* and in regional editions of major magazines, and spots on cable television stations were purchased. The theme of the promotional campaign evolved around the "new" Philadelphia Hospital Medical Center and medical advances in the four specialties.

Progress of the Product Lines

1. Cardiovascular Services. Since its establishment in the 1970s, the cardiology department had built a good reputation. The intervening years were spent developing a training program and cultivating strong referral sources, which resulted in rapid growth in the service. The infrastructure of the facility, however, had not responded to the needs the service generated by its rapid growth. Referring physicians had begun shopping among hospitals for the first available beds for their patients. To meet the volume demand and to remain competitive in terms of response time to referrals, it was necessary to open a new cardiac catheterization laboratory. To support a second lab, additional critical care beds and surgery backup, including operating room time and recovery room space, needed to be allotted to the service.

The multidisciplinary approach to the strategic planning process allowed the need for additional operating room space and staff to be identified and addressed. The process also resulted in the generation of a list of other resources needed to expand the program and a determination of their associated costs. Finally, with respect to the cardiac catheterization program, the process determined the number of new cases required to generate the revenue necessary to support the program and asked the physicians whether they could commit to attracting this increased volume. The planning process also stimulated the implementation of an outreach program to support planning for community hospital cardiac catheterization programs. Independent of the planning process, a star cardiac surgeon was recruited.

Michael Harrington, M.D., chief of cardiology, saw the process as a good one, overall. In going through the process, he was skeptical, however, that it would lead to anything. He noted: "The process served as a catalyst for getting the multidisciplinary group together. However, the same results could probably have been reached in half the number of meetings. Gaps between the meeting dates served to reduce the momentum of the projects. The effort resulted in a whole new improved relationship between nursing and the cardiology department." With respect to the marketing focus, the terminology used throughout the process, and the reference to product line management, Dr. Harrington stated, "I love the words. However, I never thought of myself as a can of peaches."

2. Geriatrics. The home health service, directed by John Irons, M.D., had a long history of success. Much of the funding for the program came from outside funding agencies to support research, patient care, and, indirectly, teaching. Dr. Irons participated in the strategic planning process as chairman of the geriatric effort. He felt that as a result of the process, the institution had only "discovered the obvious" in terms of what its "star" areas were, and that the length of time involved became rather demoralizing. Dr. Irons admitted, "I am not a big fan of strategic planning because of the period of time between planning and implementation."

3. Trauma/Critical Care. The transition from the market planning
document to the implementation plan was not an orderly process for
the trauma/critical care product line. After receiving Dr. Winthrop's
approval, the implementation plan became tangled in a political
web because of its dependence on the construction of a controversial
rooftop helipad. When asked who was currently managing the process, one senior manager listed three different individuals.

Aaron Glasser, M.D., director of PHMC's trauma center, was
acting chief of surgery at PMH during a portion of the strategic
planning process. In that capacity he was asked to participate on
the trauma/critical care market planning team. He commented,
"[Because PHMC is a Level 1 trauma center] the information concerning required resources and personnel was already present. Additionally, a large data base that supported the effective development of a market planning report existed." Many other people
agreed with Dr. Glasser that the trauma/critical care report was by
far the best organized.

After the report was submitted in January 1989, Dr. Glasser
heard that Dr. Winthrop had recommended the allocation of funds
to four areas, of which trauma/critical care was one. But, from Dr.
Glasser's perspective, he had not yet witnessed any concrete results
from the process. Dr. Glasser said, "I have not heard any direct
feedback in terms of the disposition of the proposal, and I would
be equally dismayed if activities had occurred and I was not
advised."

4. Neurosciences. It was necessary to bring together the departments of neurology, neurosurgery, and psychiatry to define the programmatic future of the neurosciences product line. One PHMC
staff member, when referring to the initiative in general, described
the relationship between the departments as the "management of a
program that has a system of transfers between services versus true
clinical integration."

The head injury program was a major focus of the neurosciences task force and one neurology representative stated, "The
neurosciences planning group is gone; it is now the head injury task
force, which is ultimately recognized as neurosurgery. It even has
its own neurologist." The head injury program also depended on

the construction of the helipad to create a truly premier program. The resolution of the helipad issue was not in the hands of the implementation team, and thus the team waited for the outcome.

5. *Cancer.* The cancer program did not meet the initial criteria for becoming an area of emphasis, as it no longer had a strong inpatient program. Yet, the hospital senior management believed that the market was there and that the hospital had a responsibility to develop and provide a high-quality program. The development of a cancer center concept, however, needed to be approached carefully, as the hospital did not want to devote a major amount of capital to the effort.

At one time, PHMC had had a large and strong cancer program. However, the clinical emphasis of the program diminished after Dr. Roy Mitchell was hired as the chief of medical oncology. Dr. Mitchell was a strong researcher, and under his leadership the clinical inpatient program dramatically decreased in size. Dr. Mitchell, who participated on the cancer market planning team, stated, "I saw the effort as an attempt to create a unified cancer program out of very dispersed and independent physician groups. The market planning meetings were finger-pointing sessions, where anger and not views were laid on the table." As a result, however, Dr. Mitchell and Dr. Murray met individually and came to some agreement. They worked with external affairs staff and developed a formal program proposal, provided to Dr. Winthrop in September 1988.

Dr. Mitchell did not receive a response from Dr. Winthrop concerning the proposal. In the spring of 1989, Dr. Mitchell was appointed as chair of the cancer care committee, a standing committee of the executive committee of the medical staff. Through a review of the by-laws, Dr. Mitchell discovered that PHMC, as a tertiary care facility, was required to have in place a unified cancer program that met the guidelines of the Joint Commission on the Accreditation of Healthcare Organizations (JCAHO). Dr. Mitchell, as chairman of the cancer care committee, then established a task force to develop and implement a unified cancer program that would meet the JCAHO guidelines.

Views of Participants

The planning process received mixed reviews from the people who participated in it. From a positive perspective, it was felt that the process provided a medium for the board of trustees and medical staff to communicate and allowed for more significant involvement of the medical staff in planning activities in general. Physician groups that had never talked to one another were seen communicating and making recommendations on issues of mutual interest.

Those who did not have favorable views of the process indicated that it only helped to discover the obvious and resulted in the loss of two critical years, during which implementation of programs would have provided the hospital with a competitive advantage. Some felt that too much time was spent in defining the logistics of the process itself, and the focus areas were hastily decided upon. It was unclear how the success of the process was being monitored with respect to increased inpatient admissions, as there was no evidence of a method for tracking the results. Some felt that the process was focused on the wrong issues and that the organization needed to strengthen its infrastructure and boast of "quick-slick operations" before it could attract a higher volume of patients. Frustration and confusion were experienced when the facilitators changed midway through the process and efforts were duplicated. Many participants felt that the communication they received was insufficient even to keep them advised of the status of the project. Following are comments of several of the people involved.

Jerry Curhan, chairman of the board of PHMC: In 1989 we anticipated that admissions to PHMC would become a critical factor, as we had to deal with cost containment issues and as we foresaw length of stay falling. We experienced our first year of running a financial loss. The strategic planning process resulted in getting the medical staff bought into five areas where PHMC could focus its resources to build our admissions. The process was necessary to get us where we are today. The medical staff reacted so well because they were such a part of it. Yet, I am sure there are some medical staff members on the "outside" who are not happy.

Gisele Rouselle (the board member who chaired the inpatient census task force): I saw the process as a method of getting the physicians to make peer decisions to determine the "haves" and the "have nots." I was surprised, given the ultimate creation of winners and losers, that I did not get a lot of flack concerning the inequity of the process. In fact, the lack of negative feedback was actually eerie. If people were not happy, this was not voiced except in particular areas that were not funded. These concerns were dealt with directly in the meetings. I did have a sense of satisfaction during the process, and ultimately everything that was recommended by the chiefs was approved and was implemented.

Dr. Edwards, chief of surgery: It was a necessary process that was made tedious and expensive in time due to the nature of the problem. It was a valuable process in that it helped to get a lot of different people together. It was an interdepartmental effort; department lines were crossed where there were common interests. It was important and absolutely necessary. We needed to make a previously subjective process objective.

The purpose of the process was not to take away independence, but rather to make the institution and individuals more productive. Initially, there was resistance to the process, as a lot of people like to be independent. Yet, there was much less suspicion at the end. If people had understood the goals thoroughly, it would have been more productive; we are now acting, in some ways, more like a business than a health care provider. Organizing by strengths was necessary; there are not many institutions that could continue to be all things to all people.

Dr. Winthrop: The process was certainly too long. What was to be a three-to-four-month process took a good year to do just the first piece of it. The other activities identified at the retreat, such as the graduate medical education program and managed care, were unable to be addressed because of the time commitment to the inpatient census task force activities. The most important outcome was a raised awareness and sense of togetherness between the medical staff, trustees, and administration. Additionally, ideas for several new programs may have spun off from the strategic planning process.

Ms. Parker, executive vice president of operations: The process worked for us. It allowed us to bring together groups to lead the organization. The best part of the process beyond the specific plans was the network of support and commitment for what we needed to do. When the market plans were submitted, it was recognized that the operational issues of implementation had not been worked on by the market planning teams. Therefore, what it amounted to was that we did the whole thing all over again. The physician chiefs passively resisted the multidepartment approach. They knew that things needed to happen. However, the change, with its elements of uncertainty, was a little threatening.

Ms. Lund, senior vice president for nursing: Initially, the perception was that it would be a fast-track decision-making process. Instead, there were a bunch of meetings with casts of thousands. The retreat did educate the group about the process, but it also served as a forum for airing ill will. I feel that we could have achieved the same ends, in terms of bringing together the players, without the long process. The effort cost us in terms of physician relations.

PHMC has a relatively high number of length of stay outliers, and our energies would have been better spent determining ways to reduce our length of stay. You cannot admit new patients if you do not have the beds.

Ms. Cox, vice president of clinical operations: The process was a valuable one due to the extent of physician involvement. It was a complicated process, however, and there were difficulties in transferring the marketing documents into the implementation phase. One disadvantage of the process was the tendency to generate false hopes and the resulting disappointments when programs were denied.

Ms. Hitch, director of health systems development: The process did bring some physicians together with the intent to build interdepartmental systems. Additionally, through the ad campaign, the identity of the institution and the specialty programs were supported. Although there were aspects of the process I thought could be modified, there was some value to the institution.

Mr. Carter, vice president for clinical operations: The retreat provided us with a think-tank process to determine which services should receive maximum benefit of our scarce resources. There was a lot of agonizing over the process because we were going to be making a public statement about which services were going to be supported for growth versus those that would remain status quo. The process did achieve the desired end result, but it took longer to complete than we had hoped. As a consequence, implementation was delayed, so we didn't get quite the jump on our competition that we had planned.

Mr. Houseman, vice president for marketing communication and public affairs: The process did result in greater participation than previous strategic planning attempts. As the process has evolved, there has not been great communication concerning the status of the programs.

Dr. Breugger, director of regional operations: The retreat served to convince the medical leadership of the need for a strategic planning process and what that would look like, and to share the truths of the environment. However, "MBA [business] terms" were used during the retreat, which ultimately offended the physicians.

The process of defining and justifying the numbers for all of the programs was agonizing. We used soft numbers in approximating expenses of the programs. This part of the process broke down as finance got involved and wanted real fiscal analysis. Since they had not been involved previously, they got real hard with the numbers, and it created a large delay in the process.

What we now have is clinical programs that have been put together. Administratively, in terms of monitoring, communication, and authority, we are not there. For one thing, we do not have the management information system required. Also, you must not overlook the difficulty inherent in people from different training effectively communicating.

Mr. Appleton's resignation provided an opportunity to alter the leadership and organization of the product line effort. Many physicians and hospital managers noted, "We could have gotten where we are now more quickly without the product line planning process." With this in mind, Dr. Winthrop wondered whether to continue with the process, alter it, or initiate a different effort. He felt that whatever changes he made should facilitate the essential efforts of analyzing and proactively responding to the changing health care environment.

Case Analysis

The product line strategic planning process at Philadelphia Hospital Medical Center had some limited success as a planning effort, consumed much time and energy, and did not substantially develop the institution's readiness or skills to implement further change. To the degree that the effort legitimized PHMC's focusing its resources on a small number of clinical programs, it was successful, although it is questionable whether it was necessary to spend so much effort to achieve this end. There is little evidence that a more flexible organization or one that is better able to deal with change resulted from the effort. No innovation appears to have been developed, nor has the level of collaboration among disciplines or departments been improved dramatically. The large amounts of time and effort expended on the planning process reinforced the negative image of the organization as one that could not change rapidly.

Prior to the product line strategic planning process, PHMC was organized functionally (number 1 on the structural continuum), although it did not have a published organization chart. It had neither integrative managers with any kind of programmatic responsibility nor any previous program-focused planning. Its previous planning processes had not provided opportunities for participation by clinicians or, for that matter, by anyone other than the vice president of external affairs and possibly a few other senior managers. The product line strategic planning efforts represent an attempt to develop both greater participation and programmatic integration. However, outcomes of both are limited. Problems are evident in the structure, selection of task force membership and leadership, perceived rewards for participants, and management of the change process.

Strategy and Structure

Located in Philadelphia, and being one of several major teaching institutions in the city, PHMC faced strong competition. Because of its location in the city, it did not have a strong outpatient service. Having neither pediatrics nor obstetrics, its primary care population was even further limited. Accordingly, the hospital sought out strong relationships with community hospitals from which it could attract tertiary care patients. To do so, faced with such strong competition, it appropriately attempted to focus its efforts on a small number of specialty programs in which it could achieve excellence and thus recognition. From a strategic perspective, this was a sound approach.

Most industries have greater flexibility than health care in the choice of products or services to offer. Yet hospitals can choose a small number of areas to develop more fully than others while providing a broad range of services. At PHMC, the hospital's relationships with the medical school and the school's need for a broad base of clinical experiences further limited the hospital's flexibility. However, in order to differentiate itself from the many other Philadelphia teaching hospitals, PHMC needed to develop areas of distinctive competence.

The medical school clinical department chairmen were chiefs at PHMC, a typical situation in teaching hospitals that are primary teaching sites for medical schools. The chiefs were quite powerful, and their needs and those of the school must not be underestimated as forces acting on the hospital and its strategic planning process. The medical school and PHMC were quite traditional. As one manager noted, "The chiefs have recognized that they have to move from individual intellectual units to economic units, but this move is not an easy one. The chiefs are actually facing a culture shock in having to face the environmental changes." Thus, it was difficult but critical that the chiefs "buy into" the strategic direction determined for PHMC.

The process described in the case initially focused on strategic planning and marketing, an orientation to product line management described in Chapter Seven. Although PHMC referred to market planning teams, in fact, by their temporary nature, these

actually were task forces (number 4 on the organizational continuum). The use of task forces is a feasible organizational alternative
for addressing the stated goals of identifying and developing "star"
programs. True teams, which serve a more permanent role than task
forces, would have been more appropriate if ongoing evaluation
and management goals were identified at the time. Involving trustees, medical staff leadership, senior administrators, and nursing
leadership was appropriate for strategic decision making—in other
words, for setting the future direction for the hospital.

The size and membership of the groups were problematic,
however. They were much too large to be effective decision-making
groups, which severely hampered their effectiveness. With sizes
ranging from fifteen in trauma/critical care and cardiovascular to
twenty-two in geriatrics, the market planning groups were too large
to attain the necessary level of participation. The literature on
group effectiveness indicates that an optimum working group is
composed of six or seven people (see, for example, Charns and
Schaefer, 1983, pp. 210–211). A greater number typically results in
excessive group efforts being devoted to managing process, which
interferes with achievement of the group's task. Group size at
PHMC is one reason the process took over two years, when it was
expected to take no more than four months.

PHMC faced a dilemma in determining task force membership. On the one hand, participation in the decision-making process contributes to people's commitment to the outcomes of that
process. Since many people—including trustees, medical leadership
and other physicians, nursing leadership, and administrators—were
key stakeholders in strategic decisions, the number of people who
needed to be involved in the group was large. On the other hand,
group size and group effectiveness are inversely related. One factor
is that large groups are difficult to schedule. For example, Dr. Harrington noted that "gaps between the meeting dates served to reduce
the momentum of the projects." Another factor is that large meetings are not very effective. One alternative to having large groups
perform all of the decision-making is to maintain the large groups
for the major policy areas (for example, the inpatient census task
force) but break into smaller, characteristically more effective working groups to perform analyses. Also, structured decision-making

techniques, such as the nominal group technique (Delbecq, Van de Ven, and Gustafson, 1975), and group process facilitators can be used to improve group effectiveness.

Even though the groups were large, they did not involve financial or operations managers to a great enough extent. They did not include finance managers at all, and operations managers' involvement was inadequate. Either the executive vice president of clinical operations, Ms. Parker, or one of the vice presidents of operations, Mr. Carter or Ms. Cox, was a member of each market planning task force. No other operations managers participated, and the senior operations managers did not coordinate task force efforts effectively with other operations managers. The finance and operations managers' inadequacy and resulting lack of commitment were apparent.

Several factors may have contributed to the limited involvement of the senior operations managers. First, they all had very broad and diverse responsibilities. Their operational responsibilities were not focused on the specific areas of activity assigned to the market planning groups. For example, although Mr. Carter had administrative responsibility for neurology, he was not on the neurosciences task force. Thus, the task forces were not areas of particular interest or effort for the senior operations managers.

Second, the senior operations managers were not responsible for the task forces. Each task force was led by a respected clinician and facilitated by a member of Mr. Appleton's external affairs division. In fact, the task forces were called market planning teams, a term that emphasized marketing rather than operations. Thus, it was easy for all of the operations to consider the effort to be "owned" and "driven" by external affairs and to feel that they were not centrally involved. Third, there appear to have been no direct efforts to engage the commitment of the operations managers, or of the senior managers of the hospital as a group, to the process. Given these factors, it could have been expected that the senior operations managers would not give the market planning task forces much attention. Consequently, when it was time to put the plans of these groups into action, support had not been garnered from either operations or finance. This necessitated development of implementation planning teams (again, technically they were task forces),

whose makeup was similar to that of the market planning groups
but with the addition of operations managers in facilitator roles and
the heavy involvement of the finance department.

Having senior operations managers as members of the marketing task forces was not sufficient to ensure their active participation. Although the senior operations managers could have
reinforced the importance of the effort, they apparently chose not
to do so, which may have reflected their low level of concern for the
process. Another possible explanation was a power struggle in the
institution. When the implementation planning task forces were
formed, it is clear that Ms. Parker took back control of the process
from Mr. Appleton by insisting that the senior operations managers
facilitate the new groups. It is not uncommon for managers to
passively resist an effort they do not control, to avoid acknowledging either another's control or the importance of the effort. By participating fully in the effort, Ms. Parker would have acknowledged
the legitimacy of Mr. Appleton's leadership and the importance of
the effort, which was introduced and driven by Mr. Appleton and
the external affairs staff. Doing so would have reduced her power
in relation to Mr. Appleton.

The lack of other operational managers' involvement in the
market planning groups cost the effort greatly in terms of getting
the operational managers on board and supportive of the task
forces' plans. Without their participation, the operational managers
felt no sense of ownership of the plans developed. Furthermore,
their skills and opinions were not solicited in the preparation of
market forecasts and cost estimates.

It is unclear whether the market planning groups had unrealistic expectations or had been given an unclear message in terms
of how far they could take their plans. Obtaining the involvement
of the operations managers in the implementation planning groups
cost PHMC momentum. By the time some of the implementation
plans were ready to be put into action, a number of people felt that
PHMC had missed opportunities in the marketplace.

Rewards

Few rewards were available for task force participation. Potential
rewards for clinicians were the resources to develop their programs,

but some clinicians questioned whether the resources were available. Dr. Winthrop appropriately stated at the retreat that money would indeed be allocated to programs that could "prove their viability." This statement implied that those who worked through the planning process would be rewarded. However, by the end of 1989, "management had decided, independently of the process, to spend $2.5 million of the $4 million allocated." This action conveyed the message that working all the way through the process was not necessary. Thus, since rewards were not contingent on participation in the planning process, a potential incentive for participation had been removed. Initially, some members of the groups might have valued establishing relationships with people from other parts of the organization. For example, multidisciplinary relationships were developed in the cardiovascular group. However, as the process dragged on without producing definitive outcomes, it eventually would have become unrewarding and frustrating.

Change Process

PHMC had a history of lack of involvement of clinical chiefs, other clinicians, and middle management in the planning process. Thus, the general understanding was that participation was not valued or expected. PHMC had to overcome these negative assumptions to move the change process forward. This required proving to people that the process resulted in positive outcomes. This could best have been accomplished by having some "small wins" early in the process, as discussed in Chapter Six. In contrast, the PHMC strategic planning process addressed a very broad agenda. The few positive results of the process were too long in coming. It was impossible to sustain momentum over this long time period when there were no significant accomplishments to show for it.

    As noted in Chapter Six, to engage clinicians' support it is important to address issues that they value and to use terminology that they understand. Neither was done correctly at PHMC. Dr. Harrington's comment—"I love the words. However, I never thought of myself as a can of peaches"—is indicative of the terminology common to the PHMC market planning process. Using such terminology and focusing on issues that are peripheral to clinicians discourages their involvement.

As a teaching institution, PHMC had paid physician leadership positions, making physician involvement on the task forces somewhat easier to obtain than it would be in a community hospital. Yet, certain medical departments were quite strong and autonomous at PHMC, and attempts at encouraging their cooperation and coordination met with little success. In some cases, the medical staff members involved understood the need for the process and were content with the results. Other physicians were incensed by the lengthiness of a process that merely resulted in plans and budgets that they believed were obviously going to come about without the strategic planning process.

At the conclusion of the effort, cases were cited of cross-departmental efforts resulting in new relationships that improved problem solving and program development. This appears to be a beneficial by-product of the task force approach. Yet, the level of collaboration that was developed was quite limited, as exemplified by the neuroscience task force having its own neurologist, rather than collaborating with the department of neurology.

At the time that the implementation plans were finalized, PHMC's management information system would not have had the ability to track the impact of new programs. Thus, there seemed to be no objective mechanism for measuring the success of the effort.

It is clear that the results of the strategic planning effort at PHMC received "mixed reviews" from those who were intimately involved and those who observed its development. It is doubtful that organizational support would have come either from the hospital or the medical staff to continue the strategic planning process or even to attempt an alternative method.

PHMC learned some basic lessons through the product line strategic planning process. Physician involvement in such an effort is ideal, but it is important for the process to be structured so that time and energy are used efficiently and so that windows of opportunity are utilized. Relations with even the physician groups that were "winners" were strained by the duration of the process, duplication of effort, and poor communication of results. Strained relations also resulted from the exclusion of operational management from the market planning process. Likewise, the duplication of effort witnessed by the planning staff, in addition to their backseat role in the implementation planning process, contributed to frustration and disharmony.

The case illustrates the strengths as well as the weaknesses of a task force approach. In addition, as in the Biscayne Hospital case in Chapter Eight, the management of the change process is a critical factor in determining the success of an innovative organizational approach.

Exhibit 9.1. Task Force Membership.

Inpatient Census Task Force

Gisele Rouselle (Chair)	Board of Trustees
Daniel Appleton	Vice President of External Affairs
Ronald Barnes, M.D.	Urology
James Black, M.D.	General Internal Medicine
Norman Carroll	Vice President of Finance
James Castle, M.D.	Associate Chief of Medicine
Stephen Cath, M.D.	Psychiatry Coordinator
Sam L. Edwards, M.D.	Chief of Surgery
John Evans, M.D.	Oncology/Hematology
Ronald Hamlich, M.D.	Director, PHMC
Richard Hayes, M.D.	Former Chief of Surgery
John Irons, M.D.	Chief of Home Health Service
William Knowles, M.D.	Director, Surgical ICU
William Lane, M.D.	Surgery
Morton Lovelace, M.D.	Chief of Psychiatry
Lee Lund, R.N.	Vice President of Nursing
Paul Martin, M.D.	Chief of Medicine
Joyce Parker	Executive Vice President of Operations
James Samuelson, M.D.	Dean, Philadelphia University School of Medicine
Bickford Sweetland, Jr.	Board of Trustees
S. Jonathan Winthrop, M.D.	President

Trauma/Critical Care

Daniel Appleton	Vice President of External Affairs
John Breugger, Ph.D.	Director, Regional Operations
Alan Cain, M.D.	Medical Director, Medflight
Sam L. Edwards, M.D.	Chief of Surgery
Richard Hayes, M.D.	Former Chief of Surgery
Edward Houseman	Director, Marketing Communications
David Gaines, M.D.	Emergency Room Medical Director
Aaron Glasser, M.D.	Director, Trauma Center

Exhibit 9.1. Task Force Membership, Cont'd.

William Knowles, M.D.	Director, Surgical ICU
Lee Lund, R.N.	Vice President of Nursing
Linda Maine, R.N.	Nursing Director
Mary Packard	Director of Planning
Joyce Parker	Executive Vice President of Operations
Jeanne Rizzo, R.N.	Senior Nursing Director
Gary Singer, M.D.	Referring Physician

Geriatrics

Daniel Appleton	Vice President of External Affairs
Donna Bailey, R.N.	Home Health Services
Paul Baxter, M.D.	Geriatrics Attending Staff
John Breugger, Ph.D.	Director, Regional Operations
Molly Cardin	Director of Social Work
Kevin Carter	Vice President of Clinical Operations
Jane Corrigan, M.D.	Neurology
Jan Daly, R.N.	Nursing Director
Katherine Hollings	Director, Physical Therapy
Edward Houseman	Director, Marketing Communications
John Irons, M.D.	Chief of Home Health Service
Morton Katz, M.D.	Chief of Staff, Jewish Memorial Hospital
Harold Lawrence, M.D.	Chief of Ophthalmology
Eileen Leband, R.N., MPH	Nursing Home Administrator
Phillip Lions, M.D.	Surgery
Lee Lund, R.N.	Vice President of Nursing
Richard Mahon, M.D.	Medicine
Paul G. Martin, M.D.	Chief of Medicine
Mary Packard	Director of Planning
George Sales, M.D.	Medicine
Bernard Tobin, M.D.	General Internal Medicine
Catherine Zolnick, M.D.	Psychiatry

Cancer

Daniel Appleton	Vice President of External Affairs
Dale Banks, M.D.	Surgery
Ronald Barnes, M.D.	Urology
Madeline Cox	Vice President of Clinical Operations
Jan Daly, R.N.	Nursing Director
John Evans, M.D.	Oncology
Martin Fineman, M.D.	Chief of Radiation Medicine
Leon Gittleman, M.D.	Chief of Pathology
Victoria Hitch	Director, Systems Development
Edward Houseman	Director, Marketing Communications
Marie Kane, M.D.	Surgery
Wayne Kingman, M.D.	General Internal Medicine
Roy Mitchell, M.D.	Chief of Medical Oncology

Exhibit 9.1. Task Force Membership, Cont'd.

Paul Murray, M.D.	Chief of Surgical Oncology
Polly Salles, R.N.	Director, Nursing Systems
Lance Wayne, M.D.	Chief of Hematology

Cardiovascular

Daniel Appleton	Vice President of External Affairs
John Breugger, Ph.D.	Director, Regional Operations
John Camden, M.D.	Codirector, Vascular Lab
Alex Carrington, M.D.	Chief of Hypertension
Donald Coles, M.D.	Chief of Pulmonary Medicine
William Green, M.D.	General Internal Medicine
Michael Harrington, M.D.	Chief of Cardiology
Richard Hayes, M.D.	Former Chief of Surgery
Edward Houseman	Director, Marketing Communications
Mary Packard	Director of Planning
Joyce Parker	Executive Vice President of Operations
A. James Richards, M.D.	Cardiothoracic Surgery
Jeanne Rizzo, R.N.	Senior Nursing Director
Harvey Saxe, M.D.	Referring Cardiologist
William Wilson, M.D.	Referring Cardiologist

Neurosciences

Daniel Appleton	Vice President of External Affairs
James Black, M.D.	General Internal Medicine
Daniel Braun	Planning Analyst
Stephen Cath, M.D.	Psychiatry Coordinator
Saul Cohen, M.D.	Medicine
Sam L. Edwards, M.D.	Chief of Surgery
Morris Fine, M.D.	Chief of Rehabilitation Medicine
Richard Fox, M.D.	Chief of Neurology
Victoria Hitch	Director, Systems Development
Edward Houseman	Director, Marketing Communications
William Knowles, M.D.	Director, Surgical ICU
Morton Lovelace, M.D.	Chief of Psychiatry
Linda Maine, R.N.	Nursing Director
Joyce Parker	Executive Vice President of Operations
David Spenser, M.D.	Neurology

Chapter Ten

Multiple Approaches
to Integration:

Hilltop Health Services

Hilltop Health Services (HHS) implemented several different approaches to integrative management, starting with "care program managers" operating in teams with nurse managers and physician leaders (number 6 on the organizational continuum shown in Figure 2.1). HHS also considered but did not implement a matrix structure (number 7), and briefly proposed operational control of programs by the care program managers, which would have implemented a modified program organization (number 8). Ultimately, integrative emphasis decreased, as HHS moved to the use of direct contact (number 3). However, HHS again was considering establishment of separate business units (numbers 8 or 9) for the "centers of excellence" that were developed from the care programs. As compared to Biscayne Hospital, in Chapter Eight, and Philadelphia Hospital Medical Center, in Chapter Nine, HHS developed stronger integrative approaches. Accordingly, HHS was able to achieve greater outcomes from its integrative efforts. The change process encountered substantial problems, however, and the roles of care program managers were never fully developed. As a result, most of the care program management effort reverted to direct contact.

HHS had several chief executives during the period covered by the case. It also had significant turnover among senior operations managers and care program managers. With each new leader came a new approach to both strategy and structure. The structural changes sometimes led and sometimes followed shifts in strategic orientation. Thus, the HHS case provides a basis for discussion of several different integrating approaches, and the relationship between structure, strategic orientation, and selection of integrative managers. To a lesser extent, it illustrates the impacts of reward and information systems and management of the change process.

As a community hospital with a voluntary medical staff, HHS faced the difficulty of obtaining participation and involvement of unpaid medical leadership. As in the teaching hospital setting, represented by the Philadelphia Hospital Medical Center in Chapter Nine, inability to involve physicians was a major constraint on the integrative effort. In contrast to PHMC, HHS did bring physicians into the process in some areas and was able to attain important accomplishments as a result.

HHS resulted from the consolidation of three independent hospitals, and a central part of its strategy was the operational consolidation of programs across the facilities and the reduction of staff and budget. Facing a competitive environment and potential loss of medical staff to its competition, HHS also had to strengthen its relationships with its medical staff. The care programs contributed to consolidation, as well as to the development of several new programs. In some areas, through program accomplishments, HHS was very successful in enhancing medical staff relationships.

Hilltop Health Services

George Vose, Ph.D., president and chief executive officer of Hilltop Health Services, was pleased to receive a certificate of need for an open-heart surgery program in the fall of 1988. This was the beginning of a true "center of excellence" in cardiology. Along with the progress, however, came the need to decide how to manage this and other centers of excellence that would follow. Dr. Vose had been considering the development of separate business units for the care programs and the promotion of the care program managers to executive director positions within the business units. As he recalled the history of the care program management effort, he wondered if it was the most effective way to structure this new endeavor.

The Setting

HHS was formed in August 1981, when Schenectady General Hospital (SGH) merged with the Ashton-Waters Medical Center. Ashton-Waters had resulted from the merger, in January 1981, of Ashton Hospital, in Schenectady, and Waters Hospital, located in Troy, New York. The primary mission of the new corporation was to "develop, improve, and maintain high-quality human health and education services for a service population of over 400,000 residents of Schenectady and Troy, New York."

Prior to the mergers, Ashton had been a municipal hospital subsidized by the City of Schenectady. Three years after the merger, Ashton Hospital was closed because of a low census. The emergency room at that facility, however, was kept open and functioned as an ambulatory care center. In early 1989, renovations had begun to convert the Ashton Hospital building into a long-term care facility. Both Waters Hospital, in Troy, New York, and Schenectady General Hospital had served their communities as general acute care facilities and continued in those roles following the mergers.

The consolidation of the three institutions was conditionally approved by the State of New York. To obtain final approval, HHS needed, within three years, to reduce its total operating budget to a point lower than the sum of the operating budgets of the three hospitals. Prior to the consolidation, the area was noted for its highly competitive health care, which had resulted in substantial duplication.

The demographics of HHS's service area reflected a disproportionately large elderly population. It was expected that by 1995, 35 percent of the population would be over seventy-five years of age. Exacerbating the situation was the lack of an influx of young people into the area.

St. Luke's Hospital represented the primary competition for HHS. St. Luke's was known as the regional cancer center. Many of the physicians in the area had privileges at both St. Luke's and HHS. During the consolidation period, some medical staff were lost to the slower-paced St. Luke's institution. HHS was also feeling pressure from a new clinic that had recently been established in the area by Albany Hospital in nearby Albany, New York.

The Organization

At the top of the Hilltop Health Services management structure was the president, George Vose, Ph.D. Reporting directly to him were Katherine Neale, executive vice president and chief operating officer, and the vice presidents of human resources, corporate development, finance, and long-term care services. The vice presidents for professional affairs, operations, and nursing reported to Ms. Neale (see Figure 10.1).

Each hospital had a director, responsible for its day-to-day operations. In addition, the hospital directors had corporate responsibilities for a number of functional departments. Each hospital also had a facility team, designed for problem-solving purposes and consisting of corporate managers and department heads of the key departments.

Figure 10.2 presents the Corporate Services Division reporting structure. In the organization structure of the corporation, some positions had corporatewide authority and others had hospital-specific authority. This required department managers who did not have corporatewide authority to report both to the director of their specific hospital and to their corporate department manager. For example, the department head of respiratory therapy at SGH reported to the SGH hospital director and to the corporate director of respiratory therapy, who was the respiratory therapy department head at Waters Hospital.

The nursing department head positions had evolved over the years as their roles broadened. Their titles ultimately were changed to "clinical chiefs." Because of the eventual cross-site responsibilities of the nursing clinical chiefs, head nurses' roles also were broad-

Figure 10.1. Hilltop Health Services, Management Structure, January 1988.

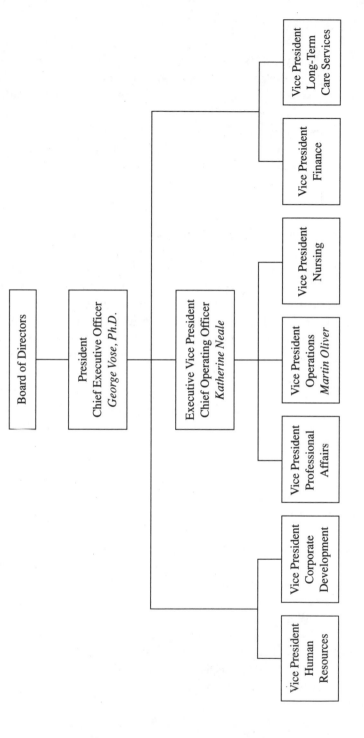

Figure 10.2. Hilltop Health Services, Corporate Services Division.

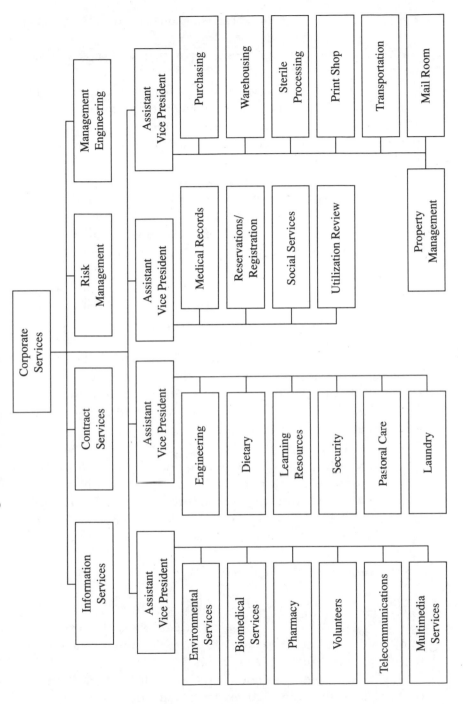

ened, and they took on traditional department head tasks, such as hiring and firing.

The patient care units were designated by specialty, although some units were more pure in designation than others. Additionally, the clinical specialties duplicated in the three original hospitals were being consolidated to individual sites. Thus, it was planned that each hospital was eventually to be recognized for particular specialties. For example, the Waters surgical program focused on neurosurgery, gynecology, ENT (ear, nose, and throat), general surgery, and some ophthalmology. At SGH, surgical specialties were orthopedic surgery, ophthalmologic surgery, plastic surgery, and some gynecology, general, and ENT surgeries were also done.

To meet the State of New York's conditions for the merger, HHS not only had to reduce the gross number of employees, but also had to consolidate and reduce the management structure of the corporation. Just after the consolidation, the management structure was "top-heavy" and attrition alone would not reduce the number of managers to an acceptable level. When Dr. Vose was hired as president, it was necessary to cut 100 full-time equivalents, and many of these were staff positions. One half of all of the nursing management positions were eliminated. The thirteen vice president positions were compressed to seven.

The medical staff of HHS was composed of a few large multispecialty groups and a few private practitioners. The medical staffs of the three hospitals were united as part of the mergers. Elected medical staff leaders were not paid for their administrative responsibilities.

The Organizational Culture

Employees viewed Dr. Vose as a highly committed and dedicated CEO. They described him as having a passion for his work and purposes that were pure. Reflecting Dr. Vose's commitment, HHS's was known as a "culture of long hours."

The local press was not always favorable to HHS. With the consolidation, the individual existence and histories of the three institutions were erased. Many people felt that HHS was not held in as high esteem as the individual institutions had been.

The two acute care hospitals that remained open had very different personalities. Waters, a teaching hospital, had an affiliation with the Saratoga Medical College. SGH had a community hospital environment. Waters was seen to have a strong nursing presence, whereas SGH was perceived to be more physician oriented and controlled. Waters Hospital was generally considered the "efficient" hospital, while SGH was regarded as the "friendly" hospital.

HHS had a large number of long-term employees, each of whom still had loyalties to one of the three original institutions. Many managers felt that this constituency of long-term employees contributed to the difficulty of changing the direction of the corporation as a whole.

Beyond the "identity crises" experienced by the individual facilities and their staffs, a major cultural revolution had taken place in terms of middle management's level of authority. Prior to 1984, all decisions were made by senior management. After 1984, there was a clear effort to push the decision-making authority down to lower levels of management; this change in management style was still evolving.

Several issues had the effect of uniting the HHS medical staffs. The rising cost of malpractice insurance, federal practice laws, and common concerns involving HHS administration contributed to the medical staffs' consolidation. Nonetheless, the medical environment was still unsettled, and the physicians felt distanced from the administration because of the complex structure of the corporation.

Sensitive credentialing and quality assurance issues, which the administration had addressed, provoked some physicians. The State of New York and the Joint Commission on the Accreditation of Healthcare Organizations (JCAHO) had increased their surveillance of quality assurance. For example, the State of New York had recently required that fractured clavicles on newborns be reported to the state. Since it was the hospital administration's responsibility to implement programs to formalize the credentialing process and sharpen the monitoring of quality assurance issues, the medical staff blamed the administration for what they saw as "Big Brother" intruding on their work. Some physicians also were angry because the consolidation of the institutions resulted in reduced bargaining power for doctors who had formerly played them off against each other.

Another source of disharmony had to do with the large number of foreign-trained physicians on the medical staff. Referral patterns among physicians reflected a distinct separation between the foreign and American medical graduates, thus adding tension to the medical environment.

Initiating Care Program Management

HHS began the implementation of the care program management effort in February 1982. The purpose of the effort was to centralize the management of the clinical services into thirteen care programs in order to eventually consolidate services within the corporation. HHS received a grant from a national foundation to develop the new management structure. In theory, care program management was supposed to apply the product line principles of industry to health care and change the focus from the individual hospital or department to the market and the patient.

The thirteen care programs were developed based on diagnosis-related groups (DRGs). In 1982, care programs were established in cardiology, mental health, and surgery. In 1983, the endocrinology, gastroenterology, medicine, maternal and child care, neuroscience, oncology, ophthalmology, orthopedics, pulmonary, and renal care programs were implemented. Six care program managers were responsible for thirteen care programs.

Selection of Care Program Managers

Many of the first care program managers hired had recently earned the master of business administration (MBA) degree from local universities. Most had no health care experience. One of the initial care program managers was a registered operating room nurse. The initial group of care program managers did not last long at HHS. Their average length of employment at HHS was about two years.

Subsequently, new care program managers had both health care experience and an advanced business degree.

Evolution of the Structure

When the care program concept was initially discussed in 1982, Bruce Ives was president of HHS. Mr. Ives was noted for his comparison of the care program management approach to the management style used by automobile and computer companies. His era of care program management was called by those involved a "straight management track."

In each care program, a team was jointly responsible for performance. The team was composed of a physician, a nurse-manager, and an MBA care program manager. The team was responsible for identifying the current and future needs of the patients served and for controlling the quality and cost of services provided. Care program management was viewed as a planning and management tool. The team was seen to have total control over its product and the resources used to provide it.

Many who were at HHS in the early days noted confusion, uncertainty, and resistance to the new management structure. Mr. Ives was described as comparing "dialysis patients to hotdogs." The MBAs' roles were not clearly defined, and many got bogged down in operational issues. Many people felt it was a time of power struggles and bewilderment.

The care program managers' reporting structure had been modified a number of times, partly to enhance its effectiveness and partly in response to changing corporate structure and attrition. Initially, half the care program managers reported to one vice president and half to another vice president. The vice presidents were also responsible for several operations departments. Vice president and assistant vice president positions for the care programs were then created. (Figure 10.3 presents the care program division under this structure.) When the vice president of care programs left the organization, the assistant vice president was promoted to vice president, and the assistant position was eliminated.

Mr. Ives left HHS in June 1983, and Steven Gross, who had worked under Mr. Ives, served as acting president. Under Mr. Gross,

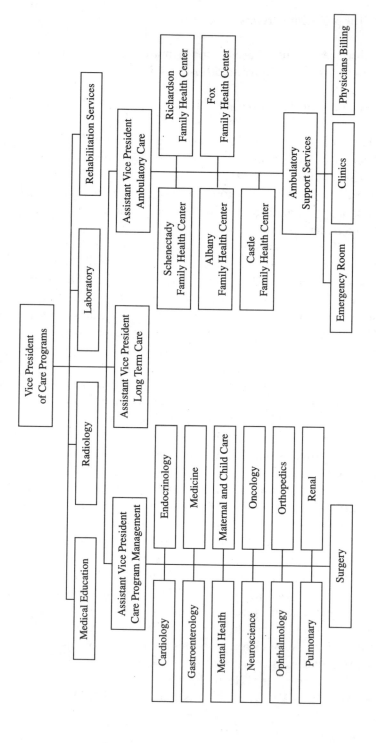

Figure 10.3. Hilltop Health Services, Care Program Division.

budgeting was to be attempted by care program. Yet, HHS never developed cost centers by care program. The nurse managers, whose roles were dramatically affected, began to wonder who their boss was and what their priorities should be: patient care management, or the gathering of statistics for planning purposes? Some nurse managers felt that the roles of the MBAs on the teams were better defined than they had been previously. In late 1983, Mr. Gross announced that the MBA would be the formal leader of each team; although this never occurred, it was reported that the nurses "went nuts."

Except in the mental health care program, nursing did not strongly support the change effort. Some managers claim that this was because of control issues; others thought it reflected a lack of understanding. Furthermore, although there were discussions about adopting a matrix organization, much of the organization apparently never fully understood the ramifications of adopting such a structure.

The physicians were described as having firmly resisted the participation of MBAs in the management of patient care, and many physicians never got seriously involved. Additionally, because elected medical leaders were not compensated, there were no incentives to increase their commitment to administrative issues. Many believed that the effort floundered because of the lack of physician support. Physicians who did participate were viewed as powerless to influence their peers.

In March of 1984, Dr. Vose was recruited to the HHS presidency. Dr. Vose, who was described as bringing to HHS a balance between business and health care, focused on long-term stability and planning. Initially, there was a conscious effort to restrain the care program managers from involvement in operational issues and to focus their efforts instead on program development and program marketing, with assistance from nursing and the physicians. This helped to further define the role of the MBAs in the care program management effort. Dr. Vose felt that the keys to success were strong nursing and the development of "centers of excellence." Each of these would be a distinct cost center, whose operations would be controlled by a care program manager working in conjunction with a physician and nurse manager.

In 1987, under Dr. Vose's direction, the care program managers were once again divided into two groups, one reporting to the executive vice president for operations, Ms. Neale, and one group reporting to the vice president for operations, Martin Oliver. It was hoped that placing the effort higher in the corporate structure would provide the care managers with organizational visibility.

In 1987, the care program managers had their own offices. By 1988, they shared office space in one large room near the corporate planning office, located at SGH.

Over the years, there had been a large turnover of care program managers. Under Dr. Vose's direction, new recruits were sought who had health care experience in addition to formal business training. Care programs were consolidated, and the number of care program managers dropped from six to four.

Dr. Vose stated his perspective on the evolution of care program management:

> With the consolidation of HHS, we recognized we needed to be in the health care versus the hospital business and not make the same myopic mistake as the railroad business had once done. We decided to differentiate the missions of the three facilities: Ashton Hospital would provide long-term care, Waters would be the high-tech regional hospital, and SGH would continue as the community general hospital.
>
> The effort started out by pursuing new programs. The consolidation took care of the structural issues, but it did not deal with operational standards. We then moved the care program managers to a more operational role in order to take care of some of the day-to-day problems. Then facilities planning became an issue, and we entered into a strategic planning process where the care program managers became heavily involved.
>
> The initial group of care program managers were unseasoned graduates; we are now resolved to using seasoned managers for the positions.

Responsibilities

In 1982, each care program manager, as part of a triad that included a physician and nurse manager, was to be responsible for resource allocation, quality evaluation, and the coordination of care that extended across departments and institutions. The team, as a unit, had authority over staffing, service scheduling, program planning, and operational and capital budgeting.

As the program evolved over the years, and with the arrival of new senior management, the responsibilities also shifted to planning and new program development. The care program managers felt that they were held accountable for the performance of a product line, its market share, and its profitability, yet they had no authority over the managers whom they needed to influence. As of the summer of 1988, a job description for the care program manager position had been in development for over one year; the care program managers perceived a lack of consensus on what their role should be.

In 1988, care program managers were involved in the development of corporate objectives. They worked with department managers to estimate volume projections for use in the operational budget, and they coordinated the acquisition of new capital items. The care program managers were generally seen as "facilitators and not leaders."

One care program manager stated that each program manager had responsibility for developing his or her line's marketing plan, but that the marketing department had full authority and control of the marketing budget and could freely alter the plan. This same manager said that 50 percent of his time was spent on planning activities, 30 percent was spent on physician and community relations, and the remaining 20 percent was spent straightening out billing problems and other, similar operational activities.

The care program managers were taken away from their specific product line responsibilities for the first four months of their tenure, under the direction of the executive vice president, to assist in the HHS master plan. The master plan, an intensive and comprehensive long-term planning effort undertaken by Dr. Vose, was developed to guide HHS through the challenging years to come in health care. The care program managers played a central role in staffing this effort.

Control of Resources

In practice, the care program managers had no direct control of the resources for their product lines, nor were they able to identify all of the care programs' uses of ancillary services. They could track charges by discharge but could not accurately relate them to costs. Budgeting by product line had yet to be achieved, and cost centers for product lines were never established.

With the eventual development of the cardiology "center of excellence," HHS needed to decide whether to break out a product line cost center and provide the care program manager with more authority and control of resources. It was expected by some that the cardiology project would serve as a pilot that would be used to determine the future of care program management.

Rewards

Schenectady County institutions competed with major industrial employers that had attractive bonus compensation programs. The care program managers participated in the same compensation program as other HHS employees: pay increases were tied to broad economic indicators. There were no performance-related bonus incentives.

Annual reviews for care program managers had been the responsibility of their immediate supervisors. One care program manager stated, however, that since there was no job description, the evaluations had become very subjective. The care program manager had had three supervisors in two years, each with different performance evaluation criteria. Performance evaluations of department managers were joint efforts coordinated by the corporate manager with input from the specific hospital director.

Information System

Early in the care program management effort, HHS entered a joint venture with the Health Systems Management group of the Yale

School of Organization and Management to develop and implement an information system designed to provide patient information by diagnosis-related groups and case mix cost accounting data. This system, called AUTOGRP, allowed the care program managers to retrieve data by type of patient more easily. Data older than two years, however, were difficult to retrieve.

The cost accounting benefits of this system were never fully realized; the State of New York was still providing per diem reimbursement, and thus cost accounting data were not useful or necessary at the time the AUTOGRP system was installed. When prospective payment was instituted by the federal government for Medicare, the institution made a decision to install a cost accounting system. This system was to be operational by January 1989. Integration of this system and the AUTOGRP system would give the care program managers direct access and ability to manipulate utilization and cost accounting data by product line.

Results

Dr. Vose felt the use of the care program management approach aided HHS in meeting some of its initial consolidation goals. Cardiac rehabilitation, mental health, maternity, and neuroscience services were centralized by the second year of the corporate consolidation. Although services were said to be consolidated two years into the effort, many claim that true consolidation, in terms of standard protocols and procedures, had only come about six years after the initial consolidation.

Additionally, a variety of clinical and support departments were centralized. To these consolidations were attributed annual budget savings of over $1.6 million. The short-term operating expense reductions were not achieved in the first two years; this was attributed to rapid inpatient volume decreases of 30 percent and to overly optimistic financial projections.

In the summer of 1988, a major achievement was realized: the acquisition of a certificate of need to develop an open-heart surgical program. It was the first such approval granted in the state in ten years. The care program manager for cardiology, Allen Cath, was widely recognized for having played a major role in the application process. Additionally, many noted that the physician involved was a proven leader and the nurse manager was highly regarded; thus, the three were seen to put together a tremendous team effort, which Dr. Vose led.

The accomplishments of the care program managers were seen primarily as program development. Many managers at HHS agreed that without the care program managers a number of the new programs would not have been achieved. The women's health program, the open-heart certificate of need, preadmission testing, equipment coordination services, increases in substance abuse capacity, and an enlarged rehabilitation program all were cited as examples of care program managers' achievements. The care program managers also successfully completed an evaluation of HHS services that included a survey of medical staff.

Some managers also attributed the increased interaction with the medical staff to the care program management structure. Others, however, complained of confusion that resulted from the unclear roles of the care program managers. All agreed that the quality of interactions and accomplishments depended on the individual care program manager. Some were highly successful in finding niches for themselves, while others never did and subsequently left the organization out of frustration.

Some department managers felt that the care program management effort limited the potential experience and exposure of department managers. Some thought that if they had been trained for it, the same accomplishments could have been achieved by department managers.

In 1982, the medical staff was said to have been highly aware of care program management and its purpose; in 1988, many indicated that the physicians would not know what you were referring to if you asked them about care program management.

Some of the care program managers of 1988 felt left out and questioned their purpose and future. Only recently had they been invited to management meetings. They had been viewed by some as an extra layer of management that at times made things tedious.

It was unclear to many where the care program management effort was going. While some saw the cardiology effort as a potential pilot program for the future of care program management and its role in supporting or leading centers of excellence, a large part of the organization expected care program management to be phased out.

Comments from Members of the Organization

Ralph Reiner, M.D., an invasive cardiologist, previously vice president of the medical staff, and an active participant on the cardiology project: Without Allen Cath, our care program manager, we would not have been able to pull together those resources required to successfully apply for the open-heart surgery certificate of need. Allen made all of the pieces come together. To keep good people like Allen, you need to give them more responsibility. I am not sure where HHS wants to go with the care program management effort. I also am not sure the system could absorb these care program managers if they were given more responsibility and authority.

Frank Gilbert, M.D., formerly president of the medical staff at SGH (just prior to the consolidation) and the first president of the combined HHS medical staff: The care program management effort has been an evolutionary process. After the consolidation, the institution began talking about a matrix management structure; it made sense, yet we never really fully understood the ramifications of a matrix structure.

The groups of physicians, nurses, and care program managers began meeting, but the process never got to function fully. I believe this was due to the significant upheaval in the early days of the consolidation. Senior managers were coming and going; all of the original people have since left. I feel we were trying to do too much all at once.

Certain programs did get consolidated, however. The care program managers played a facilitation role in these consolidations. These programmatic consolidations were influenced by circumstances such as death or retirement of older physicians and the loss of some physicians to St. Luke's Hospital.

When Dr. Vose came, things began to stabilize and HHS started to do long-range planning. The institution is much more complex than it was, and communication has become even more difficult.

The medical staff climate is somewhat unsettled. There still remains a lot of external and internal change that is threatening to the medical staff. The federal government and the state are making new demands on physicians; the hospital becomes the one that must implement these changes. The physicians feel distanced from the administration.

Katherine Neale, executive vice president of operations, and the care program managers' superior: The authority of the care program managers is the real issue. As long as there remains a separation between program development, program management, and operations management, there will be an ongoing struggle as to which party has the authority to actually make decisions and implement changes.

Where there are clearly delineated responsibilities concerning program development and operational responsibility—such as in mental health—care program management has been extremely successful. Again, in those organizations where authority and responsibility have been invested in more than one person—in other words, the separation of program development and operational management—success is far more difficult.

In terms of where we are going with care program management, I see us limiting the focus of the program managers and getting them more involved with operations through the centers of excellence concept. For example, I see the program manager for medicine becoming the executive director of our cardiac center, leading the program with a nurse manager and a physician manager, but also clearly having the responsibility and accountability for results.

Laura Bateman, corporate planner, who played a large role in the early care program management efforts: The tripartite approach, distributing equal power to the nurse, physician, and care program manager, was set up by Mr. Ives. It makes a lot of sense in a teaching hospital. But, in a community setting, where physicians are not paid for administrative positions, a huge burden was placed on them to participate. Despite this, some physicians turned out to be good leaders, while others were not so committed. Where the physician chiefs were paid—for example, in mental health—the teams worked well together.

Mr. Ives's approach had a very heavy product orientation; the physicians were referred to as "factors of production." We were talking marketing and advertising terms to the physicians; they said that they just wanted to practice medicine.

A mistake we made was starting off with too many care programs. We had planned to start off with six care programs; we initially had twenty-six. The six care program managers were spread too thin. We should have just started with a few key programs.

Additionally, there was a lot of management and physician chief turnover in the early days. The renal care program had a series of care program managers. The turnover in care program managers was partially due to the organizational confusion, but also to the lack of a career path for people in those positions.

There were also some nursing issues going on in the early days. Between 1982 and 1984, there were two vice presidents of nursing who had cross-site responsibilities. However, they each favored their own hospital. I believe they felt threatened by the care program managers, yet did not really feel they had to focus on the care program management effort. Nursing is traditionally very chain-of-command oriented.

Kim Bain, hospital director at Waters Hospital and holder of various progressive management positions at the facility: When Dr. Vose came, care program management did its thing without the previous publicity. As it has evolved, different programs are using the care program managers in different ways. Some have successfully become involved in problem solving and policy development at a more operational level. The formal authority issue has been the problem, however.

Yesterday's care program managers had a better knowledge of what was happening in the departments; today it seems to be much more a planning function with ideas on new programs. This reduced knowledge of the impact of new programs on operations is due to the ambiguity of the role. Additionally, the nursing participation in the team effort has now faded away. Nursing is now more involved with clinical issues.

In terms of where care program management may be going, I feel we need to look at the success of the cardiology program thus far. I think we will see the future of care program management get defined through the process of formalizing the cardiology effort and through the achievements of the mental health program.

We could not have brought HHS to where it is today without care program management. Examples of achievements can be cited in each of the programs. It is now evolving into the centers of excellence focus, where the care program manager has operational authority over the cost center.

Betty Taylor, clinical chief (nursing) of mental health, and an eighteen-year employee with the system: When we first consolidated, our emphasis was on cross-site issues. During the consolidation period, as we focused on systemwide issues, the quality of nursing service was on the decline.

Within one year, as care program management started, the corporation began a metamorphosis. People starting wearing pin-striped suits versus lab coats and were carrying briefcases. Meetings went from a clinical nature to looking at flipcharts with bar charts and graphs.

Stanley Ames, director of respiratory therapy: Below the department head level, people do not know that the care program managers exist. This is due to the care program managers' planning orientation. Things seem to flow better when planning and operations are kept separate.

The existence of the care program manager positions has been a tremendous time savings for department heads, and we can pay more attention to quality issues. They play a role that department managers cannot fill due to the size of operations. However, sometimes it is frustrating because we do not always hear about the issues that the physicians have discussed with the care program managers.

Mark Tosi, care program manager for mental health: I see my role as taking the lead in the planning process, data collection, interpretation, and presentation of relevant information to the mental health team. I do see my role evolving from primarily a staff function to an operational one in the form of collaborative problem solving. I do not have any formal authority and do not supervise anyone. I do not believe, however, that organizational effectiveness is necessarily associated with the use of hierarchical authority.

Carol Maxwell, care program manager for maternity and child health for two years: As care program managers, we have a great deal of responsibility yet little authority. We can draw up proposals for marketing plans or charge analyses, but we can only hope that they are accepted.

Every care program manager position is unique. I get involved in negotiating physician contracts, grant writing, representing HHS on community agencies, and project management. Care program managers want different things. Some want project management, others strategic analysis, and others want operational responsibility. This is likewise with the superiors of the care program managers. You must be able to deal with a lot of ambiguity in this position.

Jan Strong, a clinical chief: When the care program management effort was initiated, patient care was compared with assembly line manufacturing. I pictured bodies on a conveyor belt: some were traveling down the heart road. . . . What makes it so difficult for a nurse is that you learn about the patient as a whole, with physical, social, spiritual, and emotional needs. It is hard for a nurse to zero in on a heart.

The nurses still had operational problems to solve and then were asked to gather numbers. We also were forced to ask ourselves, Who is the boss? In the early days it was as if administration did not want to define the division of work. We were always stepping on each other's toes. I believe that the roles are better defined now.

The effort has been diluted. You do not hear much about it anymore. Personally, I think having a manager and a nurse for each program is a good idea. You need a manager who is close to the program who can look at it from a long-range perspective and understand the physician and technological trends.

Terry Cox, manager of budget and cost accounting: In some cases, fiscal services has had problems getting the care program managers to understand the complete financial implications of its proposals. This is primarily due to the complexity of reimbursement in the state. However, it is really dependent upon the individual; some program managers are very astute. Because of this, it is very difficult to separate the position from the person.

The care program managers who have succeeded are the ones who have learned how the institution functions and how the individual departments interrelate. The coordination of resources for new programs and the evaluation of existing programs have been achievements of the care program managers. There are certainly programs in existence now that would not have been without care program management. In these cases, the care program managers took the bull by the horns and pushed things through.

The care program managers and their ever-changing reporting relationships within the organization remind me of a play: *Six Characters in Search of an Author*. From my perspective, management has always been unsure of its role, and has tried to insert it somewhere between support services and operational management. It is always very difficult to tell where managers are currently situated because their place in the corporate structure has changed so many times over the past several years. Finance, senior management, and operations all seem to have a different perspective on their corporate role and function.

Ray Baxter, assistant vice president for diagnostics and therapeutics: Beyond mental health, the original concept never took hold. The care program managers became staffers of various projects. I suspect, however, that the effort may be going the route of cardiology, building separate budgetary units by program.

The care program managers have always been a group of nomads, bounced around, never having a leader that believed in their function. Their integration in the system was forced. They had both a lack of an administrative touchstone and lack of a defined role in the organization. In terms of who identifies with the care program managers, below the head nurse level, they are seen as just another shirt and tie.

Their success in the future is in an operational role in centers of excellence. Nursing holds the key in terms of making it work, however. The tools are being developed that include the cost accounting information system. An organizational commitment to the centers of excellence concept seems to be in the development phase.

Eventually, I believe my support departments should be selling services to the centers, as suppliers sell to customers. The skill of a support department manager is to meet the varying needs of more than one customer.

The organization has changed through all of this. You used to hear "I just cannot do it right now." Now, there is a heightened level of communication, and you more often hear "I cannot do it now, this is why, and this is when I can do it."

As Dr. Vose considered the future of HHS and the many challenges it would face, he wondered how best to use the care program managers' skills and experience. He knew the care program managers could be molded into a planning and marketing group without any authority or responsibility for operational issues. Alternatively, they could be given the operational authority necessary to totally manage their care programs. With the open-heart program moving into implementation, Dr. Vose knew he had an opportunity to move a care program manager into an important operational position. He wondered what arrangement was best for HHS—one he had considered, or an entirely different approach? With each option, he also wondered what changes would be necessary in the organization structure, power structure, and reward and information systems.

Case Analysis

With its care program management, Hilltop Health Services exemplifies an institution that over time developed several organizational forms, providing varying degrees of integrative program focus. As the visionary positions within the organization changed hands, so did the visions. The progression of institutional leaders and care program managers, the changing vision for care program management, and the modifications and evolutions of the care program managers' responsibilities and reporting relationships hindered the program's effectiveness. Care program management did yield positive results for HHS, however. These can be attributed at varying times both to the structural arrangements and to the talents of individuals. Often, success resulted from the energies and efforts of individuals who fought to succeed despite the roadblocks and gaps in the organization. The constant change and lack of consistency hindered the care program managers in finding a place in the organization and developing the influence needed for greater success. The organization structure sometimes followed HHS's strategic orientation. At other times, it appeared that the care program management effort was only whatever the organization was capable of delivering, rather than the result of a planned strategy.

On balance, care program management was seen to have contributed to consolidation and to development of new programs. These were very important to HHS's continued success. However, the uncertainty about roles, responsibilities, and power, resulting from lack of a clear plan for developing the integrating effort, took its toll on the organization. Turnover of senior management and care program managers negatively affected the care program efforts and, conversely, the ambiguity of care program management contributed to turnover. At the time of HHS's experience, however, no conceptual framework was available to assist organizations such as HHS. The prescriptions they followed, such as the pure product line management approach they initially pursued, were appropriate for only narrow applications. HHS, thus, was one of the pioneers of integrative organizational approaches.

Initial Orientation and Structure

When care program management was initiated, a major focus of HHS was consolidation of services among the previously independent institutions. This reflected a service delivery strategic orientation, which HHS often referred to as "operations" or "operational responsibility." Appropriately, the triad (nurse, physician, and care program manager) was designed for collaborative management of each care program. However, the idea was decidedly foreign and controversial in the eyes of the physicians and nurse managers involved. Its potential benefits from the nursing and medical perspectives were not made known. The effort had a business orientation that seemed increasingly necessary for the health care industry at the time, yet the language and analogies used in introducing care program management insulted the clinical professionals. Health care was compared to assembly line manufacturing, making it difficult for the clinically trained individuals to appreciate the importance and benefits of care program management. For the most part, clinicians were not drawn into and engaged in the effort, and thus the initial care program managers found themselves fighting an uphill battle with the powerful nurse manager group and the independent physicians.

As the senior management group went through major transitions, so did the care program management effort. Its focus changed from service delivery to strategic planning and marketing. Since strategic planning and marketing required less organizational integration than service delivery, the parallel organization structure, with simple direct contact by care program managers, was again appropriate to the pursuit of HHS's strategic orientation. Mental health, however, continued an effort that combined planning and marketing and service delivery, and retained its triad. This may have been a result of the insulation and specialization of that program, compared with other services offered in a community hospital.

We hypothesize that the evolution of the structure to a less integrative form (moving from position 6 to 3 on the organizational continuum) actually resulted from the lack of solidification of the triads. In 1983, HHS proposed budgeting by care program (which was not possible, given the limitations of HHS's information system), but failed to implement cost centers by program. HHS discussed the option of a matrix, while nurse managers were wondering who their boss was. Ultimately, Mr. Gross, the acting chief executive, declared the care program managers leaders of the teams. This formal declaration of care program manager authority was not only unsuccessful, it alienated and provoked the resistance of both nursing and medicine. Unable to effectively influence ongoing management of service delivery, the care program managers shifted their efforts toward planning. The organization's shift in strategic orientation, from service delivery to strategic planning and marketing, followed.

This phenomenon of strategy following structure is contrary to theory espoused in management schools, where the prescription is that structure should follow strategy. The shift in strategy occurred, however, because the structure that evolved could not support a strategic orientation that required more integration. Only the strategic planning and marketing approach could be achieved comfortably by care program managers who were striving to define and develop a role in the organization. HHS had important planning needs at the time, and the care program managers had the needed skills. The strategic planning and marketing orientation finally was confirmed by Dr. Vose, with the formal assignment of care program managers to hospitalwide planning activities.

By the time the case closed, Dr. Vose was considering restructuring into program divisions, with separate business units for different centers of excellence. We are not given enough detail to know whether these program divisions constitute a pure program organization (number 9) or whether various functions would coordinate across programs (number 8)—for example, to set and maintain professional standards. In either case, such structural change is not needed to achieve HHS's strategic objectives, and it would be difficult to gain the professional disciplines' commitment to such change. Teams are a more appropriate structure. Their failure previously at HHS was due not to the inappropriateness of the structure but to the ambiguity about roles, responsibilities, and relationships, the terminology associated with assembly line medicine, the lack of needed attention to implementation, the choice of inexperienced integrative managers, and the lack of rewards and required information to support care programs. Since HHS already has specialized patient care units, it has taken at least one major step toward dedicating staff to care programs (number 5). It can build on this to reimplement teams.

Choice of Integrative Managers

A key factor in the initial effort was the qualifications of most of the care program managers, who were recent MBA graduates with no experience in or exposure to the health care industry. They lacked credibility in the institution, as they were new, young, and inexperienced. The care program managers who fit this description had a long road ahead of them in terms of grasping the complexity of the industry, becoming familiar with the organization, and developing effective working relationships with their new management partners. Later, senior management recognized the importance of the qualifications, and more seasoned professionals were recruited.

Care program managers who established effective relationships with their corresponding medical and nursing leaders were most successful. They also appeared more comfortable operating with the ambiguity inherent in parallel structures, and did not feel the need for formal power. For example, Mark Tosi, who was the care program manager for mental health—which was one of the often-cited successes—commented, "I do not have any formal authority and do not supervise anyone. I do not believe, however, that organizational effectiveness is necessarily associated with the use of hierarchical authority."

Medical Leadership

Also hindering the effectiveness of the tripartite team, or triad, approach to care program management was the lack of stability in medical leadership. Medical staff guidelines limited physician leadership positions to one-year periods. This is commonly found in community hospitals, where physician leadership positions are unpaid and otherwise unrewarded. In each medical staff department, the leadership position is passed among the physicians and typically is seen as more of a burden than an opportunity. Performing the duties of the chief takes time away from office practice and other revenue-producing patient care activities. Incentives are lacking that would encourage physicians to stay in the leadership positions or even to sacrifice income to attend to any more than the absolute minimum of management duties. Thus, consistent medical staff participation was difficult to attain. This completely blocked the use of the triad approach and negatively affected other integrative approaches. An exception was found in the mental health group, where a paid medical director's position did exist, providing effective medical leadership and involvement in care program management. Another exception occurred in cardiology. There a medical staff member provided consistent ongoing medical leadership and support to achieve an outcome that he felt was important, despite the voluntary nature of the role and disincentives. It is important to note, however, that Dr. Vose was directly involved in the cardiology effort, and that one of its objectives, obtaining a certificate of need approval, was highly valued by the chief and other physicians.

Rewards

Neither the reward system nor the information system supported the care program management effort. The care program managers were not formally rewarded for program success. The succession of senior managers to whom the care program managers reported was dysfunctional for care program managers. Evaluations were subjective, and different supervisors had different performance criteria. They did not have a clear career path and were not included in senior management meetings. Their successes also were limited, and they were open to considerable criticism from clinicians, especially in the initial care program management effort. Thus, they had little in the way of intrinsic rewards. The members were not rewarded or recognized for cooperating with each other, and were not held jointly accountable for care program performance. Other managers were not rewarded or recognized for cooperating with the care program managers, and no sanctions were evident for not cooperating.

Information System

HHS has developed a sophisticated case mix analysis system, but, like most institutions in the mid 1980s, it was just recognizing the importance of cost accounting systems. Thus, before its cost accounting system was on line, comprehensive analysis was thwarted by lack of management information. True costs—and thus profitability by care program, DRG, diagnosis, or physician—were not possible to determine. This limitation hampered the care program managers' ability to use financial performance data for analytical purposes or to influence clinicians and other departments. Because the system was not set up to handle care programs as separate cost centers, the budgeting by care program could not be implemented.

Although charges, revenues, and utilization information could be aggregated by DRGs and groups of DRGs, these do not always correspond directly to physician groups or services, as noted in Chapter Five. Thus, there was an inconsistency in defining care programs and reporting information based on DRGs, and in managing by collaborating with specific physician groups. The lack of needed information for evaluating care program performance also negatively affected HHS's ability to provide performance feedback to care program managers.

The Change Process

Through the succession of different approaches to care program management, senior management was not clear on what it wanted the effort to achieve or how to manage it. The almost constant changes in the organization had profound effects on the acceptance and success of the care program management effort. As the case illustrates, the direct responsibility for care program management shifted many times. With each reassignment came different values, philosophies, and organizational visibility for the program. The retention of care program managers was brief. This was attributed to the confusion and level of change in the institution. The turnover among care program managers added to the organizational confusion and change. As was seen in both Biscayne Hospital, in Chapter Eight, and Philadelphia Hospital Medical Center, in Chapter Nine, the lack of senior management's understanding of and support for the integrative effort was a major factor limiting its success.

Furthermore, neither the care program managers nor senior management effectively involved nursing in the effort. Representing the largest group of professionals in the organization and being responsible for twenty-four-hour care, nursing is critical to the success of any effort involving service delivery. In reaction to the initial references to "assembly line health care," nursing did not subscribe to the effort, but saw it as antithetical to good individualized patient care. Thus, nursing did not come to the care program managers' support. Admittedly, nursing was also attempting substantial change at the time, and may have been unable to cope with more. However, collaboration between nursing and the care program managers could have been mutually beneficial.

In addition to the lack of support and rewards, noted above, indirect messages were sent to the care program managers and to the institution at large about the care program managers' status and influence. For example, even late in the care program effort, the care program managers were moved from individual offices into a large shared space, away from both the administrative suite and clinical areas. This physical move indicates a lessening of care program managers' importance and status. Similarly, their lack of involvement in senior management meetings signaled their lower level in the organization. Such minor details, even if unintentional, are often interpreted as significant messages in organizations.

External Factors

During the evolution of care program management, physicians at HHS were having to deal with external sources of change. The regulatory environment at both the state and federal levels was placing more restrictions on practicing physicians. People in administrative positions in the hospital typically had to communicate and sometimes reinforce new state or federal requirements or restrictions. This strained hospital-physician relations, further hindering the care program effort.

Accomplishments of the Care Program Effort

Although there are many criticisms of HHS's implementation of care program management, under Dr. Vose it did produce important achievements. It contributed to coordination across disciplines and across institutions. The consolidation of cross-institutional programs was accomplished, the highly coveted open-heart surgery certificate of need was attained, and other programs were developed.

These achievements were reached under adverse circumstances. The organizational complexity was greater than most institutions face, for it required managing and coordinating in three directions: across disciplines, institutions, and programs. The dual accountabilities of department managers to both their discipline head and their facility director was characteristic of a matrix structure; this introduced ambiguity, complexity, and confict. In contrast, most organizations only have to manage disciplines and programs simultaneously, and do not have the complexity of a matrix structure before introducing a third dimension. The hospitals each had different cultures and long-term employees who wanted to retain the old ways. HHS was both reducing its staff and empowering middle managers. The local press was not favorable to HHS, further complicating the change effort. The initial product line approach alienated clinicians, and that negative image of care program management carried into successive efforts. HHS's environment was both competitive and highly regulated. HHS administrators, including the care program managers, often had to carry the "bad news" from government and the JCAHO to the medical staff, which often hurt the relationship. These factors, as well as the many changes in senior management, made successful implementation of care program management a challenge. The institution did well, but could have done better. By the end of the case, with some concrete accomplishments to build upon, it is ironic that HHS does not appear to know how to proceed.

Chapter Eleven

Managing Key Factors
in a Triad Structure:

Bayview Medical Center

Bayview Medical Center (BMC) was a major teaching hospital that
effectively designed and implemented an innovative team structure
to manage its clinical services. The case illustrates, first, that the
triad structure can work effectively without one member of the
group holding ultimate responsibility and the others reporting to
that member. Many practicing managers are skeptical of an arrangement in which several people are jointly accountable and
there is no hierarchy. The BMC case shows that it can work if
several key factors are managed. Second, the case illustrates how
structure, selection of integrative managers, rewards, information
system, and change process complement each other in a successful
organizational innovation.

    Bayview had a clear and simple purpose for its effort, and
that was to be the most efficient and effective tertiary care facility
in the region in order to attract managed care contracts. The senior
managers had a vision for the future and recognized that they themselves could do no more to affect the delivery of health care than
they were doing. They believed that physicians and nurses were the

most able to manage the use of resources to provide the most effective and efficient care. Thus, a structure that decentralized decision making was developed.

Bayview's strategic orientation was clearly service delivery, with the evolutionary focus on budget and control during the period covered by the case. Bayview developed two levels of teams (number 6 on the organizational continuum shown in Figure 2.1). Three triads (or "matrix teams" or "matrices," as they were called at BMC) managed the three major clinical areas of the institution: medicine, surgery, and pediatrics. Each triad consisted of a nurse manager, a physician leader, and an administrative vice president. Additional triads managed subspecialties and patient care units. As a teaching institution, BMC had paid physician leaders, which enhanced physician participation.

Bayview's experience was a deliberately evolutionary yet disciplined approach. It was one of the early adopters of a sophisticated information system, which facilitated the challenging of then-current practice patterns. It also enabled BMC to target and measure achievements, with the responsibility for solutions decentralized to the lowest possible levels in the organization.

Much can be learned from the vision, approach, and experiences of BMC. It provides a highly successful example of innovation in health care.

Bayview Medical Center

In July of 1988, John Green, M.D., president of Bayview Medical Center, and his executive team had decided that the time had come to further the decentralization of authority to their matrix teams and to give them total responsibility for their areas' budgets. The institution was facing a $10 million deficit for the upcoming fiscal year. Measures to offset the deficit had to be taken. Given the ultimate plan to completely decentralize such responsibilities and the desire on the part of the matrix team members for budgetary responsibility, Dr. Green and his executives deliberated on the implications of making the change immediately. It would, indeed, be a true test of the power and abilities of their innovative management structure.

The Setting

Bayview Medical Center was a 500-bed not-for-profit teaching institution in San Francisco, California. Excluding obstetrics and gynecology, BMC was a full-service tertiary care facility and was the primary teaching site for Coastal University Medical School.

BMC was one of several major teaching hospitals in San Francisco. All had long been stereotyped as having particular proficiencies, reputations, and cultures. BMC considered itself the "collegial" teaching institution in the city.

One of BMC's strategies in the late 1970s had been to capture the emerging health maintenance organization (HMO) market. BMC established an individual practice association (IPA) network, formalized referral arrangements with community hospitals, and contracted with several HMOs. A second strategy of BMC was to cultivate referral relationships with physicians who had previously trained at the facility.

The Organizational Culture

Led by the charismatic and innovative Dr. Green, BMC provided a stimulating and challenging work environment for its managers and staff. An institutional focus rather than a departmental one was cultivated in the management ranks. This was reflected in the good working relationships that had been developed with physicians. High standards of performance were established for BMC managers, reflecting a heavily goal-oriented work ethic.

The executive managers of the institution believed that the necessary changes in medical practice could only be identified and accomplished by managers and practitioners closer to the actual delivery of care than themselves; thus, they believed in the decentralization of power. They also realized that the organization would benefit if influence and authority to make changes were seated in multiple levels of the institution. This was the premise used to develop the decentralized management structure they called "matrix management."

The Organization

Starting in 1983, BMC began a transition of its management structure from a traditional functional organization to the new structure, which distributed power and authority among matrix teams representing surgery, pediatrics, and medicine. Although no organizational chart of BMC's management structure existed, major reporting relationships were well known within the institution.

Reporting to the president, Dr. Green, were Donald Truman, executive vice president and chief operating officer (COO); Paul Easton, executive vice president and chief financial officer; and Sheila Thomas, chair of nursing. This group constituted the executive team at BMC. Reporting directly to Mr. Easton were the vice president of finance, Diane Pearce; the vice president for information, Ralph Rich; and the vice president of human resources, Mark Balsam.

Three vice presidents for operations reported directly to Mr. Truman. Peter Dexter was the vice president of operations for medicine, Robert Brand was the vice president of operations for surgery, and Carol Tiernan was the vice president of operations for pediatrics. Most of the ancillary and support departments reported directly to Donald Truman or through one of the three vice presidents for operations. Each vice president also was a member of the matrix team for his or her part of the organization.

In addition to other nursing functions, reporting directly to Ms. Thomas were the three vice chairs of nursing. Carol Winter was the vice chair of nursing for medicine, Laura Terry was the vice chair of nursing for surgery, and Sarah Berg was the vice chair of nursing for pediatrics. The three vice chairs also were members of their respective matrix teams.

Each of the three major medical staff departments—surgery, pediatrics, and medicine—was led by a full-time salaried chief. Two of the three medical staff departments also had a vice chairman position. The medical staff of BMC was organized under three corporations; it was far easier to deal with these entities than with more than four hundred individual physicians. Dr. Robert Rogers, vice chairman of surgery, in conjunction with Mr. Brand and Ms. Terry, constituted the surgical matrix team. Dr. Joan Singer, chief of pediatrics; Ms. Tiernan; and Ms. Berg were the pediatric matrix team. Dr. George Korman, Mr. Dexter, and Ms. Winter made up the medicine matrix team. Figure 11.1 is a graphic presentation of a portion of BMC's organization structure, highlighting the matrix teams.

To continue the decentralization of responsibility and authority, teams of nurses, physicians, and administrative managers were established on patient care units. In surgery, these teams were called DNAs, an acronym for doctor, nurse, and administrator; pediatrics called its teams UMGs, for unit management groups; and in medicine, MMTs were established, an acronym for medical management teams.

As an example of the further decentralization, the operating room (OR) was eventually restructured and cases were divided into four distinct groupings. The four operating sections were cardiac; orthopedic; general surgery, which included oncological, vascular, pediatric, plastic, and urological surgery; and head, neck, and gynecological surgery. Each surgical section had its own head nurse, and OR staff no longer rotated among specialties, as they had done previously. The booking process also was decentralized. Many people felt these arrangements contributed to improved nursing retention and a reduced orientation period. The nurses who worked in the operating room felt more like professionals; they could voice their opinions, and they would be heard.

Although no formal organizational chart existed that showed a reporting relationship between unit level teams and matrix teams, nurse managers at the unit level did report to vice chairs of nursing, and unit level administrators reported to vice presidents. Not every unit had an administrator dedicated solely to it. That is, an administrator might participate on more than one unit level team. The three matrix teams delegated responsibilities for achieving operating objectives to the unit level teams, which in turn reported back to the matrix teams.

Implementation

In 1981, BMC organized the first matrix team. Surgery was chosen for several reasons. The vice chair of surgery, Dr. Rogers, was avail-

Figure 11.1. Bayview Medical Center Matrix Teams.

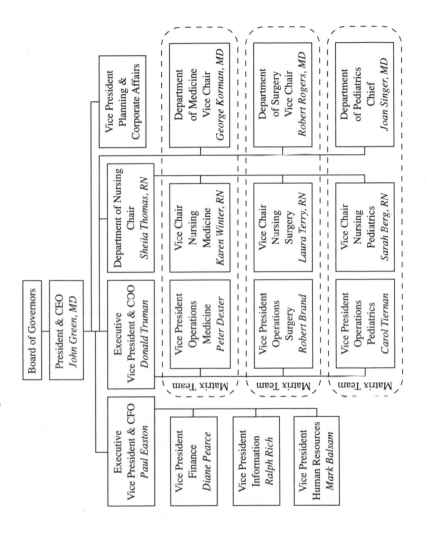

able to serve on the team and interested in doing so. Also, the surgery department tended to move quickly on new endeavors, and the executive team saw that as a positive influence on the change process. The medicine and pediatric teams were not established until a year later. Intellectual curiosity was cited as the stimulus for requests by pediatrics and medicine to shift to the matrix management model. Parallel management systems were used until all three matrices were implemented.

A formal team-building effort was undertaken for the development of the surgery matrix team. An outside consultant worked with the newly assembled team over a period of a year. As a result, ambiguity and anxiety were channeled and dealt with, and trust was developed among the three team members. Five years later, this team-building process was cited as one reason for the superior effectiveness of the surgery matrix team.

Responsibilities

When the three matrix management teams were established, they were responsible for the day-to-day operations of the specialty areas. Resource allocation quickly became a focus for the teams. For example, when the patient census for one specialty was at capacity, the matrix managers began to negotiate among themselves for additional beds from specialties that had them available. Issues that could not be resolved at this level were brought to the institution's COO, Mr. Truman. However, the matrix managers saw the need to bring things to Mr. Truman as a failure of their management abilities. This gave them further incentive to resolve problems on their own.

With the evolutionary development of the management teams at the patient unit level, these doctor-nurse-administrator teams were used to identify resource utilization reduction objectives and plans for their achievement. On a regular basis, these teams reported back to their matrix managers with information on their progress to date and problems they had encountered.

Resource utilization objectives were established at the matrix level. At the end of the fiscal year, variances were justified by the matrix teams. For the first five years, budgetary accountability had not been specifically given to the matrix managers. Traditional budgetary assignments had remained intact.

The Budgetary Process

Assigning budgetary responsibility to the matrix teams was a planned, evolutionary process, spanning a three-year period, from 1986 to 1988. Recognizing the need for information not only about departmental performance but also about specialties, DRGs, physicians, and patient types, BMC was an early purchaser of an advanced information system. During year one, cost standards per procedure for all services were developed by the finance department. This information was accessible to hospital employees and physicians through BMC's management information system. The goal for year one was to get a core group of people comfortable with utilizing the standard cost information. A policy was established to promote this: all new programs had to be analyzed and evaluated using reports from the information system.

BMC did not implement transfer pricing because there was no desire to shift revenues from one specialty area to another. It was well known that some specialties did much better financially than others; in fact, a cross-subsidization of specialties was necessary. That subsidizing took place was generally known, but senior management did not see that quantifying and disclosing it publicly was a positive motivator.

In the second year of the budgetary evolution, BMC began to link clinical data with standard cost budgeting and developed planning packages for each specialty. The information included projected volume, estimated length of stay, and standard costs per case type. There was an effort to get each matrix team to select a few case types and develop less costly approaches to care. During that year, however, the expense budget was formulated in the traditional manner, with the COO negotiating with the individual functional departments. During this time, nursing did not accept the matrix teams as sharing budgetary responsibility with them. The budgets for the clinical areas were nursing's responsibility, yet the other members of the matrix affected them.

The third year in the evolution placed the responsibility for the division budgets squarely in the hands of the matrix teams. In 1988, a $10 million deficit was projected; $4 million of this deficit was to be reduced through increased volume and productivity, and reduction in expenses. However, the institution could not "grow its way out" of the problem, and the remaining portion of the deficit would need to be achieved through other means.

The executive team members concluded that they themselves could not influence cost reductions further. They felt the only answer was to have the physicians and nurses accountable for greater cost efficiency. However, there was disagreement as to how the decentralization of budgetary responsibility should occur, as there would be significant effects on the role of the chair of nursing, Ms. Thomas.

As the areas of fiscal responsibility evolved, more attention was given to costs per unit of service. For the first few years of the structure, ancillary departments may not have noticed any difference in terms of how the institution was managed. As the financial picture dimmed, however, it was expected that pressure would be applied on the ancillary departments to reduce their unit costs.

Matrix team members believed that the transfer of financial responsibility would also bring about the transfer of the traditional administrative and medical staff problems of resource management. It was expected that the matrix teams would soon be the ones who had to say no.

Power

One reason for adopting the matrix structure was to decentralize power and authority in the institution to allow for more effective and efficient responses to the changing health care environment. By grouping the three major constituencies of the institution—the medical staff, nursing, and administration—effective problem solving could occur. The united fronts developed by each matrix team, a by-product of the change, proved to be extremely powerful. When the members of a matrix team reached agreement on a given issue, they felt that there was no stopping them.

By design, the power at the matrix level was intended to be equal among the three members of the team. However, in practice, depending on the issue at hand, one member would have more influence than the others. There was evidence that physicians in matrix teams tried to dominate, but few cases were recalled of this dominance compromising the integrity of the groups' professionalism.

The Selection of Integrative Managers

In developing the matrix teams, the executive group paid a good deal of attention to who the individual members were and how the chemistry among them would develop. If one member of a matrix needed to be replaced, the executive group allowed the remaining matrix team members to select the replacement. Their perceived success was seen as a function of the people chosen to fill the matrix team roles.

Within the matrix teams, mutual respect for one another and for respective professions developed. The often-quoted statement "If you need something, act as a team" reflected the incentive for and reinforcement of the matrix team concept and the development of cohesive, productive relationships among the disciplines.

The vice presidents for operations were seen as the key members of the teams in that they needed to be able to work with the nurse and physician members. All three people in those positions had previously been directors of planning.

Case Management

BMC implemented a case management system as a formal means of monitoring quality and cost of care. Case management plans were developed by the teams at the patient unit level to serve as standardized plans of care for specific case types. Patient goals and outcomes, planned nursing and medical interventions, and actual and potential patient problems having a high probability of occurrence made up the case management plans. "Critical pathways" were developed as abbreviated versions of the total plan.

Each patient was assigned a case manager, typically that patient's primary nurse. The case manager coordinated the delivery of care provided by the "collaborative group practice," which included other nursing care givers and the patient's physicians. The case management plan was shared with the collaborative group practice and the patient so that each member of the group was aware of any potential problems and anticipated outcomes. At various times during that patient's hospitalization, the case was reviewed and compared to the patient's care plan in order to keep the delivery of care effective and efficient. Established goals of continuity of care, patient outcome, length of stay, and resource utilization were achieved. Additionally, a high level of nursing satisfaction and professional development was attributed to the case management effort.

Information System

BMC had long been recognized as a leader in aggressively applying information technology. It was one of the first hospitals to install a sophisticated system with the capability of integrating financial and clinical data, which could be accessed at different levels within the organization for different purposes. Specialized modules supported both department managers, who needed standard costing and cost control, and case managers, who needed to monitor utilization of resources. Each matrix team had the financial and utilization information needed to monitor its specialty and pinpoint problems. Various modeling applications were designed to support the budgeting process and other simulation activities. This allowed investigation of implications for resources for both the specialty and for functional departments when services were being implemented, changed, or discontinued. Integrated financial and clinical data could be accessed at any level of detail desired; for example, they could be aggregated by patient, by physician, by patient care unit, or by specialty. The concurrent nature of available reports generated by the system allowed for timely case management.

Results

Agreement was consistent that the institution could increase its efficiency through the development and application of protocols for case types, and that its ability to solve problems and ensure coordination had increased. There was good evidence, for example, of reduced length of stay for specific case types. Quality of care was enhanced by means of the standard case management plans and effective collaboration between medicine and nursing. Able to offer competitive fixed prices to HMOs, BMC's volume increased dramatically.

Decentralization of problem solving down to the unit level allowed primary nurses greater exposure to and understanding of the goals of the organization. Information sharing was seen to have improved along with cross-departmental problem solving. Improved attitudes among the nursing staff were witnessed, as they felt they had greater control by being responsible for developing the case management plans in conjunction with the physicians. Nursing in general no longer felt that it was fighting its battles alone; support from the medical staff and the administration was provided through the matrix structure. One consequence of the teamwork was an increase in time required of team members. For example, it was no longer solely a nursing decision to hire new head nurses; other members of the matrix team had to take time to be involved in the decision.

Tension remained, however, between the old and new ways of doing things. The chair of nursing, Ms. Thomas, had to develop a new role for herself when decision making was pushed down in the organization. In addition, several people felt that BMC was just one step away from splitting the nursing department among the three specialties, eliminating the need for a centralized nursing department. Furthermore, pay inequities existed between the administrative and nursing representatives of the matrix teams. When the total responsibility for budgeting was given to the matrix teams, this became a heated issue.

Views of the Participants

John Green, president: My personal goal is to create a cutting-edge health care environment with physicians and nurses as managers. This is based on my belief that physicians and nurses are the ultimate managers in health care.

When I first came to BMC, we began working on a number of control system problems, such as billing issues, and we were able to gain a lot of points politically. I then got everyone to agree to a goal of ambitious growth. I strongly believe that reality is better than reputation; some institutions are seen as the emperor, but in reality their clothes are tattered and torn.

The beginning of matrix management occurred with our interest in offering fixed prices to HMOs. Between the information system and the knowledge of physicians and nurses, we could predict resource use for patient types. Fixed prices for cases should attract volume; it worked in cardiology, where we went from 250 to 1,000 cases per year between 1981 and 1988. I see this as good business, but more important, it is good patient care.

Donald Truman, executive vice president and chief operating officer: The issue at the time we implemented what I call the "modified matrix structure" was that of resource utilization and its impact on the cost of care. It was clear that Paul [Easton], John [Green], and I could not influence costs through utilization. We could not mandate a 5 percent reduction in lab tests ordered. We needed to have the physicians and nurses responsible for making changes.

As finances get tougher, it is important for the matrix teams to have a broader corporate focus. Our goal is to have physicians and nurses thinking more like managers, and vice versa. This leads to understanding each other's perspectives better and making better decisions.

The key issue for me is choosing the right people for the roles. There has to be a chemistry there.

Sheila Thomas, chair of nursing: When the matrix teams were created, my role changed a lot. I had to let the vice chairs of nursing do their job. My job was to support them and to keep their focus on a unified philosophy and central goals for the nursing department. Tasks such as dealing with grievances, hiring head nurses, and staffing in general had to get more decentralized. Things have developed to the point where I am comfortable with the vice chairs running their matrices.

The disadvantage of the matrix management approach from a nursing perspective is that it takes more time. Nursing now has to be more concerned with all of the issues, and you end up spending a lot of time away from purely nursing issues. Additionally, you just cannot talk collaboration—you have to be committed to it. The end result, however, is much better. We have not had to fight budget battles alone.

Laura Terry, vice chair of nursing in surgery: It had been decided to experiment with a new organizational structure, and it was observed that if it could succeed in surgery, it could succeed anywhere. We chose to begin with a long-standing project, preadmission testing—one that the hospital had long been wanting to implement. We met with great success.

We use each other to cut across the professional lines. One key to our success is having an operationally oriented physician as part of the team. We are all equal in terms of the authority in our role. Yet, we joke that one of us is more equal than the others.

Robert Rogers, M.D., vice chair for surgery and the physician member of the surgery matrix team: The relationship of the surgical matrix has been evolving. The underlying theme is for the differing organizational power structures to learn from one another, as we each have our own sets of codes and interests. It has taken several years to develop the trust that is needed.

I believe the decentralization of authority can lead to increased flexibility and more rapid responses to the environment. Yet, we currently have only gone about 75 percent of the way along the decentralization continuum. The budgeting process still occurs centrally. I would like to see the budgeting process be totally delegated to the matrices. Yet, there always will be a need for someone to have an organizational focus to balance institutional priorities.

Robert Brand, vice president for operations in surgery: The surgical matrix has effectively created a recognition of the importance of acting as a team. If you need something important, act as a team. It has been proven that you cannot stop something that has the support of administration, nursing, and physicians.

The first couple of requests made to the executive office were the hardest. Now, it is easy. When we need something, we get it. We do not have to fight for everything. In fact, now the executive office comes to us and asks, "What do you need?" There is a sense of trust that has developed between our matrix and Donald Truman. He knows when we cannot give any more.

For the first four or five years, the ancillary departments were not impacted dramatically by the matrix system. They were not sensitive to the effort to use less resources. We do, however, have the authority to go outside BMC for services if we are not satisfied. We are now starting to see a decentralization of ancillary services. For example, we put the blood gas function in the operating room.

Peter Dexter, vice president for operations in medicine: Our matrix structure has helped us most specifically with the reduction in costs per case. We have been able to increase the organizational efficiency through the development of standardized protocols of care and by eliminating the delays in the system. In terms of impact on patient care, there is currently no scientific answer, but patients can get in and out quicker, without delays. They also receive new home health services. It tends to promote a "complete person" perspective of care. There also appears to be an improved attitude among staff, as they feel they are more in control.

George Korman, M.D., vice chair of medicine and the physician member of the medical matrix team: The major reason for changing the organizational structure was to increase the administrative responsibility on the part of the medical staff. Obviously, the motivation to change grew from the acknowledgment that use of resources was controlled by the physicians, versus administration. It has proven to be a very powerful tool; the people who could make it happen were all there.

With the strength of our information system and case management, we have a much better fix on how resources are being used and can ensure the appropriate utilization. Our plan is to go to the HMOs with fixed prices for care provided to specific types of patients.

Carol Winter, vice chair of nursing for medicine: With the implementation of the case management effort, nursing was responsible not only for patient outcomes but also for the fiscal viability of the hospital. What makes it difficult is that cost effectiveness has not been a part of the educational curriculum of physicians and nurses.

When we were interested in trying case management, no one said, "This is what you must do." Rather, we pondered aloud, "I wonder what they are doing in other places." In 1985, we asked all the head nurses to work with their physicians to develop one case management plan for a particular case type. We now have over 140 case management plans. If you talk with physicians individually, they like the case management system. In groups, physicians will not admit to it. Through case management, physicians know exactly who is responsible for their patients. Additionally, case management makes patients very secure. Each nurse the patient sees knows what is happening in the other areas where the patient is receiving care. The critical path of targeted activities and achievement is shared with the patient.

Carol Tiernan, vice president for operations in pediatrics: The group practice concept in pediatrics, where nurses and physicians on patient units set goals for patient types, has really worked well. We have been able to get them aware of the information available and the need to monitor utilization. The group practice concept has really been a helpful mechanism to achieve a better bottom line. Eventually, I see the need to reward the physicians in some way for meeting the targeted goals.

The institution is good at working with physicians. We are sensitive to when to push. A lot of what we have been able to accomplish is really due to the people and not the system. Human nature is involved. The structure alone cannot do it all. People's strengths and weaknesses will affect the success of the effort.

Diane Pearce, vice president for finance: Our approach to decentralizing financial management and encouraging the use of the information system has been an evolutionary one. We believe if you do something radical in a short period of time, you will lose the organization. We used incentives to encourage people to learn how to use the information system. For example, physicians who were requesting to start new programs were required to use the information system's reports to verify the program's viability.

The flexibility of our information system has enabled us to make cost center managers more sensitive to their costs. We have been able to start new programs without increasing our costs and actually have brought prices down from the high end to the low end of the range [for hospitals in the city]. Enthusiasm for what we can do, however, has not penetrated beyond the top two or three tiers in the organization—and it needs to happen.

James Miller, administrative manager for the operating room: With the matrix structure, you truly see a balance of interest and collaboration. The intent is to put the nursing, physician, and administrative concerns on equal footing and to create the best possible program for the patient. The matrix approach results in a three-way bond. The only disadvantage is that the equal footing sometimes gets tilted. It really depends on the individuals involved.

Dr. Green is a pretty exciting guy. He has defined a roadmap for the organization. It keeps changing, but we move and really try to get things done. I think that the people who work here really enjoy the challenge.

Mark Balsam, vice president for human resources: Our evolution from the traditional to the matrix structure is a long-term process. It is clear that people in a traditional functional organization do not have the incentives to ask the questions that are necessary today. Only a collaborative team can make this happen.

People nowadays do not want to be just cogs in a wheel; they want a voice. We need to design jobs that are meaningful enough and that allow people to feel that they have their say. From this, they reap great rewards. Smart organizations will give people a real role in making decisions. And the best decisions are made at the lowest level. This is where the "keys to the kingdom" lie.

We are still in the process of solidifying our hybrid matrix structure. We have a very traditional nursing department, but at the same time we have some more contemporary forms. There is, however, a lot of tension between the old and new ways of doing things.

Case Analysis

Bayview Medical Center (BMC) is an excellent example of an organization that has effectively implemented a set of integrative arrangements, including structure, rewards, selection of integrative managers, and information system, to pursue its organizational strategy. Although several steps remain in its change process, BMC has done well with its implementation to date. In terms of both organizational arrangements and the change process, BMC provides, for the most part, a prototype of an innovative hospital that has effectively managed a balanced, evolutionary approach to change.

Strategy and Structure

As is the case with many large medical centers, BMC faced a highly competitive environment. In contrast to PHMC, which focused its strategic planning efforts on selecting a few areas to develop (see Chapter Nine), BMC's strategy was to differentiate itself from its competition by being a highly efficient provider of a broad spectrum of patient care and contracting at fixed prices to HMOs and other managed care providers. To achieve long-term effectiveness, BMC could not just promote an image of excellence; it had to actually provide the services efficiently and effectively.

BMC's senior managers recognized that they could not mandate efficiencies in patient care delivery and that they had to involve and empower physicians and nurses to achieve that objective. Given a strategic orientation that focused on service delivery, it is appropriate that BMC developed a team structure to manage its major services (number 6 on the organizational continuum shown in Figure 2.1), with additional teams at the patient care unit level. BMC involved the three major components of the organization in its teams: medical leadership, nursing leadership, and administration. The teams provided the vehicle for collaborative management of both the major services and the operations of units. They involved senior people in all three disciplines who could make the decisions required of them. In addition, this indicated to the rest of the organization the commitment to this approach.

Although they used the terms *matrix* and *matrix teams*, their structure actually was a team parallel structure, as described in Chapter Two. The primary reporting relationships of the members of the matrix teams were to their functional departments (medicine, nursing, and administration, respectively). While maintaining the functional reporting relationships, the teams were developed and empowered to make decisions regarding their clinical services.

Structurally, BMC does not need to shift the reporting relationships any further. They are attaining nearly all of the potential advantages of collaboration and focus on management of the clinical services, as described in Chapter Two. Altering reporting relationships to develop equal authority of the functional departments and the clinical services, which would result in a true matrix structure (number 7), is unnecessary. It would add organizational overhead without significant advantages. Going even further, into the range on the continuum where the clinical service reporting relationships are primary (numbers 8 and 9), is inappropriate. Although BMC could increase the focus on management of its clinical services by further altering its structure, little is to be gained, and further change would weaken the functional departments substantially. For example, changing to a structural form further to the right on the organizational continuum would weaken the influence of the nursing department. As discussed in Chapter Two, this risks long-term weakening of professional development and professional standards and practices. It is less likely, for example, that BMC's nurses would have implemented case management throughout the institution had they been organized exclusively by clinical specialties (if structure number 9 had been adopted). This would be true even if they had retained a "dotted line" relationship to a nurse executive (number 8).

The teams can be strengthened through other organizational mechanisms than altering the structure. Primary among these are the information system, budgeting, and personnel evaluation based on performance of the clinical services. BMC senior management was considering whether to decentralize additional budget authority to the teams. This is an appropriate action to take, as it places responsibility for management of the financial aspect of the clinical service at the level where the most relevant information is available. This will enhance the teams' ability to affect resource utilization. Lacking at the time of the case, however, was a practice of holding the functional departments accountable for the cost per unit of their intermediate products (see Chapter Five) or giving the teams greater influence over the functional departments. With its information system, BMC is positioned to increase the accountability of both teams and functional departments. BMC was approaching these decisions cautiously, however, as it did not wish to encourage harmful competition among teams or between teams and functional departments.

It also should be noted that the team structure has not extended to other departments or to other than three clinical services. To the extent that nursing, medicine, and administration are the primary disciplines, BMC is achieving much of the potential collaboration, and it is not necessary to involve others directly in the teams managing the clinical services. Little information was provided about dedicating personnel in other departments to care for patients of particular clinical services. To the extent that consistent assignment is attained, greater collaboration in actual delivery of services can be achieved. Although it is not necessary with the team structure to have every service represented by teams, an appropriate next step for BMC is to consider where additional teams could be effective.

Selection of Integrative Managers and Team Membership

In contrast to community hospitals, teaching hospitals such as BMC have full-time paid medical leadership. The full-time positions, physicians' admission of patients to the single facility, and economic incentives that are different from those in community hospitals have facilitated the involvement of medical leadership in the teams. These leaders, the chairs and associate chairs of the clinical departments, are the primary vehicle for influencing the practice of other physicians. Without their involvement, the teams' potential would be severely limited, as was seen at Hilltop Health Services (Chapter Ten).

Nursing leadership, also, functions as a partner in the teams. This contrasts with having nursing report to an integrative manager who is either the medical leader or the administrative manager. The three disciplines work as equals, so none of them is lower in status than the others. Nursing as a profession has been working hard to further develop its professional position. Nursing is responsible for most of the twenty-four-hour patient care. It is best for both the profession and the institution that nursing have the status and formal responsibility to function in partnership with medicine and administration.

At BMC the nursing department appears to be in a strong political position. This is indicated by job titles and by nursing's ability to implement case management well ahead of most other hospitals. "Chair of nursing" and "associate chair" are academic titles that convey a parity with the medical staff structure. Even so, this case study reveals some tension between nursing and the team structure. Tension is inherent in these arrangements because team needs and departmental needs are in some degree of conflict. In addition, as exemplified in nursing, senior managers often experience discomfort when their subordinates are empowered, for it brings their own responsibilities into question. The key issue is not whether conflict exists; it is how well conflict is managed.

Finally, the selection of the administrative members of the teams is significant. First, they were high-status, credible individuals. They brought their personal credibility and relationships to the new and evolving positions. This is in sharp contrast to the cases of Biscayne Hospital and Hilltop Health Services (Chapters Eight and Ten). Second, at BMC the administrative members of the teams all had backgrounds in planning. The planning skills clearly were important in the early phases of the teams' activities. Additionally, the planning, or staff, orientation may have alleviated the tendency of the administrative managers to feel the need for line responsibility to control the teams.

Rewards

Intrinsic incentives of the structure encouraged the matrix teams to resolve issues at their level; having to take issues to the executive office was seen as failure. This norm rewarded the team members for effective problem solving among themselves. For example, the matrix teams successfully negotiated with one another to reallocate beds when the census in one service was climbing while that of another was falling. In addition, with an information system capable of reporting performance in their areas, the matrix teams were able to obtain feedback on their performance. The rewards inherent in success are the most powerful motivators available in organizations.

Intrinsic rewards were augmented with goal setting and support from senior management. The level of trust developed between the teams and Donald Truman, the chief operating officer, was quite high, and contrasts with the relationships between integrative managers and senior management in all of the cases in the previous chapters.

As the change was implemented, the teams' successes were acknowledged and they were given further responsibilities. It is important to note that behavior consistent with the change process was rewarded, sending signals to the participants and others that the new behaviors were desired. Two critical examples were rewarding the teams for developing agreement and presenting a united front to senior management, and requiring physicians to use data from the information system to support their requests. Had senior management allowed members of a team to promote their self-interests, rather than encouraging them to focus on the joint interest of the team, the teams would not have succeeded. Had they "ordered" physicians to use the information system, it is more likely they would have developed greater resistance to change than adaptation of behavior.

The reward system for team members was soon to be in a state of flux, however, as the nursing team members were interested in receiving compensation equal to that of their administrative counterparts. It is important to note that salary inequities could upset the balance and interfere with the level of trust and teamwork in the integrative teams. This should be a red flag for BMC.

Information System

BMC's information system was a critical factor in its success. It had installed one of the most sophisticated systems available. The system's capabilities allowed tracking of utilization, expenses, and revenue needed for managing both departments and specialties. Many organizations have the same hardware and software as BMC. What distinguishes BMC from other hospitals is its ability to use the system effectively as a clinical and management tool.

The Change Process

The change effort at BMC is clearly an example of success. Much of this success can be attributed to the development and communication of a vision by Dr. Green, the support by the senior managers, and the attention given to managing the evolutionary change process.

BMC began the change process in surgery, where there was both interest in the new approach and a good chance for success. BMC started with a project, preadmission testing, that was recognized as important and that could yield "wins." After success in surgery, BMC moved into implementation in the other two services. Through its team-building efforts, BMC also recognized that trust and collaboration cannot be developed overnight, and that professional facilitation could aid their development. Over a period of five years, we see the development of high levels of collaboration.

The change process did take a long time. BMC had the time available, as it was not in a situation requiring a quick turnaround. BMC could evolve incrementally, building on successes as it moved forward, and integrating changes into its reward and information systems while further developing collaborative relationships. When it reached a financial crisis in terms of the projected $10 million deficit, BMC had in place a powerful mechanism to address it. BMC's change process contrasts sharply with Biscayne Hospital's (Chapter Eight), in terms of both time and results. In comparing the change processes at BMC and PHMC (Chapter Nine), it is clear that just allowing enough time is not sufficient to achieve successful change. BMC's change process was conservative but continually moved forward.

Several people felt that the success of the organization in bringing about innovation resulted more from the people involved than the organization structure itself. We argue that it was a combination of structure, systems, and people reinforcing each other at BMC. Mutual respect among team members, among teams, and between each team and senior management was evident. The organization realized that people want to feel involved and influential, and BMC provided opportunities whenever possible. Although anticipation of the change evoked some anxiety within the organization, challenges to the health care industry were generally recognized, and the executive office's sensible efforts to meet them head on inspired enthusiasm, confidence, and excitement.

With its blend of structure, information and reward systems, selection of integrative managers, and management of the change process, BMC achieved significant improvements in financial and clinical performance. Its accomplishments were attained while its strengths were maintained and its professional disciplines, such as nursing, were enhanced. This positioned BMC well for future success.

Chapter Twelve

Strengths and Disadvantages
of a Service Line Structure:

Hanna–Thorndike Hospital

The case of Hanna-Thorndike Hospital (HTH) illustrates both the advantages and the disadvantages of structuring into a program organization (number 8 on the organizational continuum shown in Figure 2.1). Each program division was termed a "service line" and was the responsibility of an executive director. Nursing staff were organized by service line, with all nursing in a service line being the responsibility of the service line nursing director. Nursing directors reported to executive directors of their service lines. Only a dotted-line relationship remained with the nurse executive. This case presents both the practical and emotional implications of this kind of structural relationship.

HTH was pursuing a combination of all three strategic orientations. Planning and marketing, budget and control, and service delivery were all elements of the responsibilities of the executive directors.

In addition to the service line program organization, the case highlights the linkages to the medical staff, organization of ancillary and support departments, and the implications of the feedback

258

and rewards given to the executive directors for their service lines' performance. The HTH case also exemplifies the effective management of a change process.

Hanna-Thorndike Hospital

Barbara Donaldson, R.N., M.S.N., president of the 540-bed Hanna-Thorndike Hospital, wondered whether it was time to alter the hospital's innovative service line management structure and return to a more traditional one. By mid 1989, it was obvious that prospective payment had caught up with the progressive institution, and the trend of financial losses was threatening its future. The hospital's length of stay had been creeping up as a result of increased patient acuity, along with a rising percentage of Medicare and Medicaid patients. The hospital's emphasis on productivity and budget reductions had not been sufficient to stem the losses, nor had utilization management efforts made a major impact.

The Setting

The current organizational configuration of the Boston, Massachusetts, institution was a result of a 1985 affiliation and eventual merger of two independent hospitals: Hanna and Thorndike. HTH was one of the first hospitals to reorganize into a corporate structure. In 1984, Hanna Corporation was established, and Hanna Hospital became a subsidiary of The Hanna Corporation (THC). Ralph Nagle, who was often referred to as the "guru" of Hanna, was then the chief executive officer of HTH. Following Mr. Nagle's resignation in 1985, Keith Smith was hired as CEO of THC. Mr. Smith formed the vision of THC as the premier multihospital system in Eastern Massachusetts.

With the impending merger with Thorndike Hospital, which was planned to be the first of many hospitals that would be attracted into the THC system, the functions of human resources, support services, and finance were centralized at the corporate level within THC. This superstructure was designed to support the large multi-institutional system that was envisioned to eventually compete with Massachusetts Health Plan.

*Implementation and Evolution of
the Organization Structure*

In 1985, THC was faced with the need to physically merge the
Thorndike and Hanna operations. Concurrently, THC recognized
the challenge of maintaining quality patient care and healthy financial performance in the face of increasing competition, reduced
rates of payment, and declining utilization of services. In response,
THC leadership took the opportunity to restructure the organization into service lines. A presentation to hospital management
groups noted the following reasons for restructuring into service
lines:

1. Service line management increases accountability of hospital
    managers for (a) patient and physician satisfaction, and (b)
    bottom-line results.
2. Service line management thus provides strong incentives for
    maintaining or improving both quality and continuity of pa-
    tient care in the hospital setting.
3. Service line management creates an organizational focus de-
    signed to make the hospital both more sensitive and more re-
    sponsive to changing marketplace interests and concerns.

    THC undertook a year-long planning effort to implement
service lines. It outlined the following objectives for service line
management:

A. Financial
    •   Achieve greater accountability for profits and losses
    •   Be more responsive to changes in reimbursement
B. Organizational
    •   Establish greater decision-making authority at the level
        closest to patient flow, and for the individuals most knowl-
        edgeable about services
    •   Provide structure and incentives supportive of creative
        management
    •   Eliminate management layers
    •   Encourage greater partnership with physicians

C. Services
- Be more responsive to competitive forces
- Be more customer driven and patient oriented
- Enhance the clinical management of patient care

D. Planning and development
- Ensure greater control of strategic resource allocation by individuals holding operational responsibilities
- Build a management structure that will result in synergy between programs
- Provide a clearer delineation of resources within the organization

The plan was to establish independent service lines as profit centers and groom "mini-CEOs," who would have total authority over their service lines. To symbolize the service line managers' power and authority, the title "executive director" was chosen. Most service lines had, in addition to the service line executive director, a medical director and a nursing director. Some service lines directly controlled specific nursing units and ancillaries used exclusively or predominantly by the service line. As of June 1985, eight service lines and five support departments were delineated (see Figure 12.1). The eight service lines included the following:

- Mental health services
- Women's and infants' services
- Rehabilitation/neuroscience/orthopedics services
- Respiratory services
- Cardiac/vascular services
- Oncology services
- General medical/surgical services
- Older adult services

In 1988, the rehabilitation/neuroscience/orthopedics service line was combined with the older adult service line, and a new emergency services line was established.

To incorporate the service line management concept into the affiliated Hanna and Thorndike hospitals' structures, Ms. Donaldson, who was president of Hanna Hospital, was given the respon-

Figure 12.1. Hanna-Thorndike Hospital.

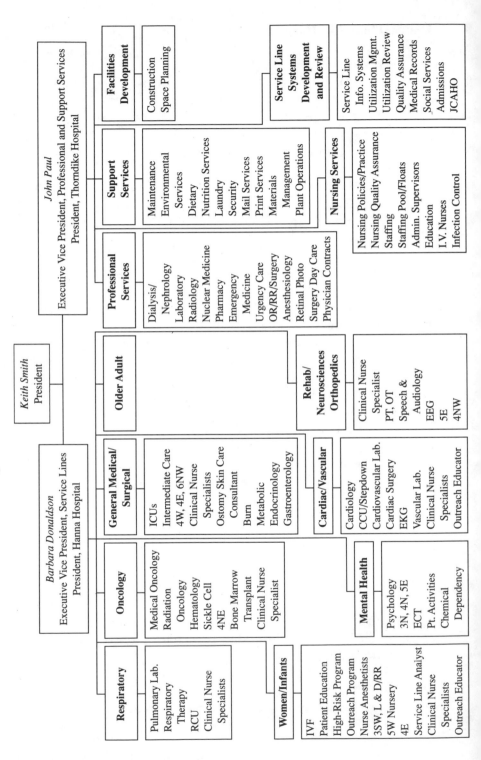

Hanna-Thorndike Hospital

sibility for service lines and the additional title of executi
president for service lines. Concurrently, the president of Thor.
Hospital, John Paul, was given additional responsibility as ex
tive vice president for professional and support services. Both I
Donaldson and Mr. Paul reported directly to Mr. Smith.

Nursing Services

To give the executive directors direct line authority, the central
department of nursing was split; nursing directors and clinical
nurse specialists reported to the service line executive directors. A
central nursing services office was maintained for purposes of staffing, nursing education and development, infection control, and
nursing quality assurance.

The decision to split the nursing division was a painful one,
as there was much resistance from nursing. The administrators responsible for the decision spent much time and effort convincing
concerned staff nurses and managers that the new organization
structure would meet the needs of their patients, the requirements
of regulatory bodies, and the professional development of their specialty areas.

To combat the resistance against decentralization of the nursing function, a nursing leadership council was established. This
group was led by the nurse executive and was composed of the
nursing directors, clinical nurse specialists, and other nursing administration personnel. The leadership council, which met once a
month, was the governing body for nursing practice issues as well
as the place for general policy and procedure development, planned
program implementation, and collegial interaction.

The central nursing office that remained after the reorganization was considered a "safe" place for nursing directors to go for advice and support. Many felt that the central nursing office had become
the mediator between the executive directors and the nursing directors
on some issues, and both were noted to seek counsel there.

Ancillary Services

Wherever possible, ancillary services that primarily supported one
service line were placed organizationally within that service line. For

ysical therapy, occupational therapy, and speech and
were part of the rehabilitation/neuroscience/orthopedics
ie. However, departments that served many if not all service
mained centralized. These centralized departments tended to
ie support to the service lines in such a way that support staff
me somewhat dedicated. For example, environmental services
ff had designated areas of coverage. Decision support staff were
divided into teams that concentrated their energies on specific service
lines in the areas of budget, cost accounting, planning, marketing,
financial analysis, and management engineering.

Selection of Service Line Executive Directors

The eight executive directors were recruited in March 1986, with six
of the eight coming from within the HTH organization. For some
of the service lines, the appointment of the executive director was
a natural transition. For example, the nurse managers for the
general medical/surgical and maternity and infant care areas were
promoted to executive directors for those service lines.

Role of the Executive Directors

Ultimately, the service line executive directors were responsible for
the overall operations of their service lines. Revenues, expenses, and
service line productivity were the major concerns of these executive
directors. Their principal accountabilities included the following:

- Ensuring provision of high quality care
- Monitoring and maintaining fiscal viability according to agreed
  upon standards
- Maintaining long-term viability through program development
  and marketing
- Maintaining appropriate contracts and relationships with the
  medical staff
- Ensuring quality of care through quality assurance activities
- Coordinating activities with the other service lines
- Enhancing long-term viability and competitive advantage of the
  service line

In addition to fiscal responsibilities for the departments under its domain, each service line was designated a specific set of DRGs by which success was measured. In some cases, the unit where a patient in a particular DRG eventually received care was not the responsibility of the service line executive director charged with that particular DRG. It was felt that this blurred, if not confused, accountability.

For each specialty area, the executive director was viewed as the administrative representative. Executive directors were seen as the advocates for their services and responsible for facilitating the determination and obtaining required resources to provide a cost effective and quality service. The job description for the executive director position called for the provision of administrative direction to medical, nursing, and clinical managers in the development of objectives, standards of care, and policies and procedures. Interdepartmental problem solving typically was the responsibility of the executive directors. In terms of program development, the executive director was responsible for strategic planning, market plan development, and monitoring consumer satisfaction and quality of care.

The executive directors had the authority in regard to expenditures and program development, as approved in their business plans. Executive directors were required to consult their superiors about policy decisions that would affect the total organization, and about expenditures and plans not outlined in the approved business plans.

The executive directors were responsible for hiring and developing personnel within their service lines. However, the nursing director of a given service line was delegated the authority of hiring, firing, and evaluating nursing personnel. Additionally, nursing directors were typically delegated the authority to approve expense requests within their budgets, and authority in regard to productivity and quality assurance.

Medical Leadership

Medical leadership varied among service lines. For some, a traditional medical director position existed. The service lines of mental health, rehabilitation, and emergency services were examples of this. For others, such as general medical/surgical services and women's and infants' services, it was difficult to appoint one medical leader, and the executive director and nursing directors had to work with different groups of physicians, depending on the issue at hand. Thus, some service lines had a more formal relationship with the physicians providing service to the patients than did others.

Information System and Support

When HTH changed to a service line management organization, its information system did not have the flexibility needed to provide hard data for service line decision making. Accounting in terms of service line profitability was available but was utilized only on an annual basis. Budgeting according to anticipated resource use was not possible; consequently, the executive directors had difficulty in monitoring actual versus budgeted resource use.

A major initiative of HTH was productivity management. Each department was expected to maintain an average productivity level, over a two-week period, of 102 percent. Engineered standards were developed for each department, and reports generated by decision support staff assisted the executive directors and, specifically, their managers in monitoring the productivity level of their departments.

Even though initially the organization envisioned having service lines negotiating and contracting for services from support departments and with the ability to go outside the HTH organization if satisfaction for the service was not achieved, it was not anticipated that service line management would go to this extreme. The decision support group did not foresee charging back, for example, the services of housekeeping and food services to a service line.

Assessment of Service Line Management

An advantage clearly recognized throughout the organization was the availability of administrative support and advocacy by specialty. Many people felt that access to administration was improved, which contributed to greater distribution of information, more focus on the needs of individual departments, and a good base for physician linkages. Members of the organization felt that there was a more comprehensive understanding of the needs of their consumers, better program planning and implementation, and a more effective focus on quality of care. As one physician noted, "We now have an advocate versus an obstacle in administration."

Many people felt that no other structure made much sense for some of the service lines. The structure of the women's and infants' service line was appreciated by both the hospital staff and the medical staff, as it allowed the service line the flexibility and responsiveness to truly cater to their clientele.

Some of the disadvantages attributed to the service line effort concerned fragmentation of the organization. Some people thought that individual service lines focused on their own needs without any apparent regard for the organization as a whole. For example, when the cardiac care unit offered double time to its staff nurses in order to cover staffing on off-shifts, the intensive care nurses gained leverage to demand the same compensation. When the pharmacy raised its prices to improve its profitability, other service lines that used these pharmaceuticals, and could not pass on the increased costs, saw their financial performance erode.

Issues that were common throughout the organization were difficult to identify, and many found themselves duplicating the efforts of their peers in other service lines. Collaborative relations between service lines were encouraged, but as the competition for hospital resources increased, the cooperative spirit waned.

About half of the executive directors employed in 1989 had either nursing or other clinical backgrounds consistent with their service line specialties. The other half had backgrounds in industrial engineering, business, or public health. Some people in the organization felt that clinical experience and credibility were critical for the success of an executive director. From this vantage point, nursing directors shared the frustration and time commitment involved in having to explain technical issues thoroughly to the nonclinical executive directors. Beyond the language barrier, some people indicated that staff nurses and nurse managers no longer felt supported, and that decision making within the structure required more meetings.

Others, however, felt there was a sense of challenge and
respect for the nonclinical executive directors. The relationship that
evolved between the executive directors and their managers was seen
as valuable. Nursing directors who preferred this alternative explained that they had moved away from the emotionalism and protection of nursing, and more creative problem solving was a result.
Additionally, the information that nursing directors received was
generally viewed as more abundant and relevant under the new
system. A by-product was that nursing no longer had to fight its
battles alone; there were many people who would advocate for the
cause.

Comments from Members of the Organization

Sharon Irwin, director of decision support: We are just now beginning to be able to provide the executive directors with the information that they need on an ongoing basis to understand and act
on profitability. The stumbling block in the whole picture is that
you cannot hold the service line executive directors accountable for
what physicians will or will not do. If we could lick this, we would
have it made. It is not even management by consensus. If the physicians do not want to change their practice, they won't.

Jack Ornstein, executive director of support services: The attitude
here is that we want collaborative competition—not cutthroat competition. As financial pressures become worse, however, the conflicts are increasing, and there are a lot of personality conflicts
among the executive directors.

   The group expectation is that you'll do what's best for the
hospital. It's a fine line that's hard to achieve. We're lucky the group
works well together, but as resources shrink, conflicts increase.

   It is important to know what the service line versus the vice
president level is accountable for and has authority for. An ongoing
conflict is nursing quality assurance. Is this a central nursing function or a service line function? This is yet to be defined.

   The executive directors are very good at advocating for their
areas in terms of articulating their needs. Yet the current limits on
authority undermine their ability to be effective.

Anne Cox, nursing director of mental health services: Breaking up the nursing department has been extremely difficult. The support system and camaraderie of the traditional structure just is not there. Yet, it has helped to move me away from traditional thinking and the emotionalism and protectiveness of the nursing profession. Although my superior and I do not always speak the same language, we do work together to come up with more creative resolutions.

Service line management seems to be too expensive, as there are more top administrative managers and a need for more meetings than I have ever seen. I would go back to the traditional structure in a minute.

One bone of contention is the fact that I am evaluated based on my patients' length of stay, which is something that I have no control over. I am accountable for this, yet I do not have the authority, not to mention the time, to influence length of stay.

Dena Paris, R.N., M.S.N., nursing director, oncology: The biggest problem with service line [management] for me personally is that there is competition with everything not cancer-related. We used to meet as a group of head nurses around a common foe—sometimes helper—the director of nursing. There are a lot of similar problems on units. Meeting as a group gave us power. What service line management did was isolate me—and I had been here six years already when it came in. So you really were on your own. We met, but it was very different. The message was competition. What we got, others didn't, and vice versa.

As originally presented, we'd have our own dietary, housekeeping, and marketing. It never happened. It was bull _____ .

Ruth Wright, R.N., assistant director, cardiac care unit (CCU) and intermediate care unit (ICU): The structure and purpose of service lines has divided nursing into segments. You lose the feeling of one big happy family.

We work under a system of nursing hours per patient day, based on acuity. If you have a patient who takes management nursing hours—one who's combative, loud, or difficult—you need a "sitter." You have no hours for that, so you don't want that patient on your floor. You try to move the person to another floor, whether the patient has the particular disease process for that floor or not. It's most likely that med/surg units try to keep these patients in CCU, ICU, or ITC.

Bob Sales, R.N., medical/surgical service line executive director: Med/surg was a potpourri of what didn't fit logically elsewhere. I also feel schizophrenic about the service line and nursing units. The service line is defined by DRGs. Surgery is defined narrowly by a set of surgical DRGs. Similarly, medicine and medical subspecialties are narrowly defined. The schizophrenic part is that at first I didn't have control over the units and labs where care to my patients is delivered. For example, in GI [gastrointestinal], I didn't have responsibility for the endoscopy center, but most of my program is done there. Most of that has been remedied now.

In my mind I've developed as a "support service line." I have patients in my own service line and provide support for other service lines. That helps people in the service line see the impact on other service lines. They are so interrelated, you can't say, "They're not my patients."

I was the one raising questions the loudest when we considered changing to this structure. Really, nursing hasn't lost, but has gained. Before, there was one vice president of nursing with four or five other vice presidents. Now there are eight service line executive directors who have come to realize the importance of nursing in delivering their service—eight voicing the interest of nursing.

The service lines have enhanced program planning and focused people's view of it. We developed the cardiac surgery program when we were in the functional structure, just evolving into service lines. I was the nursing director responsible only for the CCU. We had representatives for the OR, for the cardiologists, for surgery—there was always someone missing when we had our planning meeting. When we transitioned to service lines, Jim [Short] had all the pieces of the cardiac/vascular program except for the OR. There are very clear differences under the two systems.

There's not a good relation between measurable objective performance in the service line and our compensation. We have had poor data systems and don't know how we are doing financially.

So we are held accountable on productivity measurement and expenses.

We don't control the discharge planner. You take the social worker assigned. If you don't like that, you have to influence the social work department.

Jim Short, executive director, cardiac/vascular services: A year and a half ago, I formed a committee to reduce length of stay. Dr. Parker and I chair it. It includes a cardiac surgeon, cardiologists, nurse managers, surgery managers, anesthesiologist, clinical nurse specialist, and one person from Utilization Management. . . . We revised standing orders to reduce the use of ancillary services, substantially reduced blood use for cardiac surgery, and decreased length of stay. . . . In making changes, you have to prove to the doctors that patient care won't suffer. It may take six months, but the momentum of the group will carry.

Henry Parker, cardiologist: The change to service line worked out quite well for us. It unified the Cardiology Department, CCU, and cath lab. It aided program development and utilization management. It let us get angioplasty and cardiac surgery off the ground.

To have a successful cardiac surgery program, you need volume. We heard there were cardiologists at a MetroWest hospital who were not happy. They didn't have a voice in administration. Here there is a cardiac/vascular administrator they could identify to hear them out. Jim Short courted them. He had the same goal as we did. The service line concept has let that happen.

Ms. Donaldson's Decision

The cost of operating a service line management organization was felt, by some, to be a burden in terms of the added management positions required. Additionally, it was difficult for most to know whether they felt service line management had been successful thus far. With many changes in the management structure and the damaging payer mix shifts, it was impossible to determine the contribution of service line management to the financial health of HTH. With the looming potential for subsequent modifications to the organization structure, some people felt it was necessary to limit further change and maintain the current structure in order to sustain the confidence of physicians.

Ms. Donaldson now had to decide whether the innovative service line management structure could guide HTH back to a strong fiscal position or whether the structure had become a liability and needed to be changed.

Case Analysis

Hanna-Thorndike Hospital changed its structure into program divisions called service lines and altered reporting relationships so that nursing directors reported to service line executive directors, rather than to a central nursing department. A dotted-line relationship existed between the nursing directors and the nurse executive, and the nursing council served as a mechanism to coordinate nursing issues across the service lines. These elements identify the HTH structure as position number 8 on the organizational continuum. The fact that all departments have not been reorganized similarly to nursing clouds the categorization of the organization on the structural continuum. In practice, however, few departments other than nursing are large enough to be fragmented. Thus, the HTH organization comes about as close to being a prototypical number 8 as any hospital does, and it provides an excellent example of both the benefits and problems with these arrangements.

Structure

Many benefits of the program organization were realized at HTH. Its approach included all three strategic orientations described in Chapter Seven. HTH was able to achieve a focus on market segments, better identify costs and utilization, and implement improved service delivery. For example, the case describes several positive outcomes in the cardiac/vascular service line. The recruitment of a new group of cardiologists was attributed directly to the responsiveness of the service line executive director. HTH also effectively achieved a reduction in length of stay and in blood use for cardiac surgery.

Many nursing directors also noted the benefits of the service line arrangements. They felt they received more relevant information and that "nursing no longer had to fight its battles alone." Based on the theoretical framework presented in earlier chapters, it is expected that improved collaboration within service lines will occur. This would facilitate operations within each service line, with the accomplishments contributing to satisfaction of nursing directors, executive directors, physicians, and others involved in the efforts.

In addition, for each clinical area, the service line executive director provided a responsive point of access to administration. As is characteristic of the program organization structure, service line executive directors at HTH were able to make resource commitments. The empowerment of divisional managers—in this case, the executive directors—is an important element of a program organization. It is possible because division managers by design have both an overview and control of their whole "business." Also, observe the contrast between the influence of the executive directors in HTH and the product line managers at Biscayne Hospital (Chapter Eight), PHMC (Chapter Nine), and Hilltop Health Services (Chapter Ten). Only at Bayview Medical Center (Chapter Eleven) does the level of influence of the triads even approach the influence of executive directors at HTH. The executive directors not only had an interest in how their service lines functioned, they also had the authority to make decisions and respond to opportunities and concerns. Thus, many people, including physicians, saw that they had "an advocate versus an obstacle in administration."

The structure had inherent disadvantages, however. First, by fragmenting the nursing department, coordination among the various divisions of nursing was impaired. As organizational mechanisms, the nursing council and dotted-line relationship to the director of nursing simply are not as strong as a direct reporting relationship and being part of the same whole department. This is expressed in various ways. For example, Dena Paris, the nursing director in oncology, noted, "There are a lot of similar problems on units. Meeting as a group [of head nurses] gave us power. What service line management did was isolate me—and I had been here six years already when it came in. So you really were on your own.

We met, but it was very different." Ruth Wright, assistant director of the cardiac care unit and intermediate care unit, said, "The structure and purpose of service lines has divided nursing into segments. You lose the feeling of one big happy family."

Hospital managers in general, and those at HTH in particular, should be concerned about fragmenting nursing and other departments, as this removes the organization's vehicle for professional development, maintaining professional standards, and generally advocating for the professions. It is easier to coordinate around concrete service delivery issues than around the more abstract issues of "professional development." Already problems in coordination among parts of nursing are evident; in the long term, the negative effects on the hospital will be increasingly significant. Without a nursing identity, HTH risks becoming perceived as a place that is not supportive of the profession and not a good place to work. All organizations have to maintain professional competence. They all have to coordinate among disciplines. Any organization structured into divisions experiences fragmentation among those divisions. Such structural issues are not unique to health care.

What is unique to health care is the position of physicians not having formal reporting relationships into a hospital's hierarchy. At HTH, the medical staff is not formally linked into the service line structure. For example, the medical staff does not report to the service line executive directors, nor do the directors report to the physician leadership. Where collaboration has been achieved, as in cardiology, it has been done through development of the personal relationships between the service line executive director and/or the nursing director and physicians. In this regard, the HTH service lines operate as informal teams and are more dependent on the development of relationships than on the formal authority of the executive directors. Where there are several specialties in a service line, with many physicians and no single physician leader, it is much more difficult to establish relationships between nursing management and physicians and between executive directors and physicians. This was exemplified by the medical/surgical service line. Also, HTH determined service lines by both medical specialty and DRGs. Since these two did not always correspond, executive directors sometimes did not have control over portions of the organization where patients of "their" physicians were receiving care.

Finally, the internal organization of departments to dedicate staff to particular service lines, as in decision support and environmental services, facilitated coordination between the support departments and service lines. This internal reorganization represents position number 4 on the organizational continuum, and provides a basis for much of the coordination attained even without changing formal reporting relationships. Where staff were not dedicated to service lines, such as in dietary, housekeeping, and marketing, coordination and responsiveness were not as effective.

Considering both the positive and negative aspects of the structural arrangements at HTH, the hospital is experiencing more of the disadvantages than is necessary to reap most of the benefits it currently derives. If a team structure were utilized, it would provide a focus and contact in administration, yielding the types of advantages evident in the cardiac/vascular service line. Coordination in teams or task forces to address particular issues, such as reducing blood utilization for surgeries, does not depend on the formal authority of the service line executive director. It is dependent on the integrative manager's having the credibility and interpersonal skills to involve the important stakeholders in discussion and action to address the issues. A similar argument can be made for the other positive outcomes from the service line arrangements. That is, they could be attained nearly as well with teams as with the total restructuring into service lines. The major difference is that without the change in formal reporting relationships, the integrative managers do not have the benefit of the formal authority. This is most helpful initially, when they are in the process of establishing their credibility. Once the integrative managers have shown their worth, the formal authority is less important than their competence-based influence, especially to clinicians.

Other Structural Arrangements

As noted above, departments other than nursing have not been fragmented and similarly brought into the various service lines. Instead, two different approaches were taken. In one approach, whole departments were moved to report to individual service lines. For example, physical therapy, occupational therapy, and speech and audiology became part of rehabilitation/neuroscience/orthopedics services. To the extent that patient care needs focus the activity of these disciplines in the single service line, this reporting relationship is beneficial. The disciplines, as part of the service line, become more responsive to the service line's needs. Ultimately, the integrative manager can determine resource allocation, staffing, and even personnel decisions for those disciplines that are part of the service line. This provides for greater control and decisions more attuned to the needs of the service line.

There are, however, negative aspects to incorporating disciplines into service lines. To the degree that the disciplines become responsive to the needs of their service lines, their focus is shifted away from the overall needs of the total hospital. Their primary mission becomes meeting the needs of their service lines, and their secondary mission becomes serving other service lines and the rest of the hospital. Bob Sales's comment, "At first I didn't have control over the units and labs where care to my patients is delivered," exemplifies the problem with the arrangement of having patients cared for by parts of the organization controlled by other service lines. To put the issue quite bluntly, the department managers know where their bread is buttered and respond appropriately. The hospitalwide focus of these disciplines is lost when they are part of one service line. Some realignment was done at HTH, as is evidenced by Bob Sales's comment, "Most of that has been remedied now"; but, no matter what service line a given discipline is placed in, the discipline will not have the same organizationwide focus it would have as an independent department. The more a discipline needs to balance its efforts across service lines, the greater the problem with its being placed in any single service line.

As an alternative approach, HTH placed several disciplines and functions under the professional services service line in the Professional and Support Services Division. In that it does not generate revenues as the other service lines do, it is not the same kind of organizational entity. In fact, HTH may have called it a "service line" only to maintain a uniform approach and consistent emphasis on the service line concept. This arrangement does allow more of an organizationwide focus than the arrangement described above. It is not clear, however, why all of the functions in professional services are in that part of the organization. Why, for example, are surgery day care and anesthesiology in professional services rather than in general medical/surgical services, and, more important, where should they be? This can be answered by examining the interdependencies among these services and other parts of the organization. To the extent that they serve other service lines, such as cardiac/vascular and orthopedics, they are appropriately placed under professional services. To the extent, however, that they primarily serve medical/surgical patients, they should be part of that service line.

Rewards and Information

To reinforce the structural arrangements and give executive directors more authority, HTH senior management delegated substantial decision-making discretion to the service lines. In addition, service line financial performance and productivity were monitored. This performance measurement clearly got managers' attention and focused their motivation. However, the dysfunctional aspects of the narrow focus also were evident. The measurement system was encouraging managers to optimize their service lines' performance to the detriment of the total hospital. Examples include the cardiac care unit's offering double time to its nursing staff, without considering the implications for other areas of the hospital; the pharmacy's raising its prices; and units' attempting to transfer patients based not on patients' clinical needs but on the effect on productivity measurement. As discussed in Chapters Four and Five, focusing behavior through measurement and rewards has the positive effects of increasing motivation to attain performance goals but the negative side-effect of narrowly focusing behavior. Both are evident at HTH.

The components of the professional services service line provide supportive elements to the clinical service lines. In other words, they provide "intermediate products," as discussed in Chapter Five. Therefore, since they do not produce final products or associated revenues, it is more appropriate to measure their performance and hold them accountable for costs and quality of services, rather than for profitability. If HTH had done so, it is unlikely that the pharmacy would have unilaterally raised its prices, for it would not have been motivated by profit performance.

The Change Process

HTH did effectively implement the new arrangements. It appears to have been sensitive to issues of communication, and it did address many of the concerns of clinicians. HTH chose respected nurses for many service line executive director positions. This helped to alleviate some of the negative implications of fragmenting the nursing department. HTH achieved several "wins" that reinforced the change and contributed to its momentum. With the degree of change implemented, HTH can be called "innovative." Thus, in contrast to Biscayne Hospital and PHMC, where ineffective change processes blocked innovation, HTH managed its change process effectively.

HTH demonstrates the most radical hospital reorganization of the cases presented in this book. It is one of only a small number of hospitals to have implemented a program organization. This structure, however, is a more radical realignment than is needed to achieve HTH's objectives. HTH's performance measurement system amplifies some of the advantages of the structure, but also the disadvantages. The organization is now fragmented by service lines, rather than by disciplines. HTH is close to achieving an arrangement of several "mini-hospitals," each managed by a "mini-CEO." They share a common building but not the same organizational goals. As they compete against each other over time, the dysfunctional aspects of their organizational arrangements will become even more apparent.

Chapter Thirteen

Implementing an Integrative Structure:

Waller Memorial Hospital

Waller Memorial Hospital was a community hospital with a fairly conservative corporate culture. Over several years, through an evolutionary process, it implemented first task forces and then a team approach to integrative management. The hospital sought both improved patient care and increased market share. Thus, its primary strategic orientations were service delivery and planning and marketing. As it increased its emphasis on ongoing management of service delivery, the hospital's development of teams was appropriate.

The primary focus of the Waller case is on the process of implementing an integrative structure. Thus, more information is provided in this chapter than in previous cases on how the hospital developed the new structure. Since the process and content of change are highly interrelated, information on structure, selection of integrative managers, rewards, and information system also is presented in the case and discussed in the analysis.

The senior management group was highly involved and committed to making the effort a success. This was critical both to supporting the integrative managers and to the overall change process. To take advantage of their clinical competency, physician relations, and earned influence within the organization, clinical managers at Waller were promoted to integrative management positions and referred to as "service line managers." In some cases, these individuals also maintained their functional management positions.

Physician involvement and support, although difficult to achieve, were seen as keys to success. Recognizing the importance of medical staff involvement, Waller management developed strategies for achieving it early in the implementation process.

Waller illustrates many important aspects of implementing an innovative structure. Although it did experience some difficulties and did not achieve all of its objectives, overall Waller was highly successful. The case and analysis illustrate many of the elements of managing change discussed in Chapter Six.

Waller Memorial Hospital

Richard G. Tracy, president of Waller Memorial Hospital, reflected on the achievements of the service line management effort that had been in place in his institution for the past two years. He was pleased with the problem-solving capabilities of the service lines as well as the positive relationships that had developed between the hospital and the medical staff. As part of the hospital's strategic planning process, Mr. Tracy pondered the expansion of the service line management approach to support other service areas and even smaller programs.

The Setting

Waller Memorial Hospital was the single hospital in a Northwestern city of 32,000 people. The institution had developed a strong image in the community and the region as a high-quality institution. The hospital's strategy for survival had been to continue its development as a regional referral center for certain specialties, even though this approach often conflicted with the hospital's maintaining its community hospital demeanor and charm.

Reflecting the work ethic and values of its leader, Waller's culture centered around a standard of excellence achieved by hard work, dedication, and caring. The focus on what was best for the patient was pervasive at all levels of the institution. This value drove the hardworking management and staff.

Through Mr. Tracy's leadership, the hospital often initiated collaborative efforts with other hospitals in the region to acquire expensive technology. Mobile lithotripsy and magnetic resonance imaging were two examples of efforts that were developed to serve several institutions in the surrounding area.

The Medical Staff Environment

The medical staff had grown rapidly over the previous five years and boasted a fairly comprehensive range of specialties and subspecialties and a high percentage of board certified physicians. The medical staff included the large multispecialty Roberts Clinic, with the balance being independent practitioners and small single-specialty group practices.

Prior to the mid 1980s, the medical staff environment was one of cooperation, respect, and friendly competition. Many informal agreements were made among competing specialists. In the mid 1980s, as the pressures of prepaid and managed care became more acute in the region, the medical staff initially worked together as a whole to determine the best route for the community. To the surprise of many, the Roberts Clinic suddenly broke off discussions and affiliated with a larger multispecialty clinic that itself was affiliated with the region's tertiary care facility. This affiliation ultimately led to the Roberts Clinic's relationship with an existing prepaid health plan that served the region to the south of Waller.

Shortly after the Roberts Clinic developed its new affiliation, the independent physicians in the community formed an independent prepaid health maintenance organization. Thus, a gap between the two factions of the medical staff was created, and the real political and competitive complexities within the medical community began to emerge. Over the years to come, the clinic built on its strong base of primary care physicians and recruited many of its own specialists in areas not previously provided within the clinic. The clinic's need to refer to the independent physicians decreased.

Turf that had once been protected by a handshake had now become open game.

Investigation of Product Line Management

Waller began to investigate the benefits and potential fit of product line management in 1987. Management was oriented to the concept and purpose through seminars and tracking of relevant literature. In 1988, all senior managers and department heads attended a nationally conducted seminar held at the hospital.

Lois Glenham, then in a staff position to Mr. Tracy, was given the responsibility of proposing an approach to the senior management group, generally referred to as the administrative team. Intensely interested in the experiences of other health care institutions that had committed to product line management, Ms. Glenham visited a variety of such sites. Through her meetings with people at each of the sites, Ms. Glenham learned that product line management was used for many different reasons and that the organization structures used to carry out the approach were just as varied. Through this assessment of the experiences of others, it became clear that it was necessary to tailor the use of product line management to Waller, based on its intended goals and culture.

The Service Line Management Approach

Ms. Glenham consulted with Waller's administrative team to determine its key reasons for wanting a service line approach. Administrators placed major emphasis on the need to ensure top-quality patient care by understanding the needs of the "customers," whether they be patients, families, physicians, the business community, or the community at large; improving interdepartmental coordination and communication; and integrating the medical staff into problem solving and planning. The administrative team felt strongly that focusing on the improvement of quality through these means would positively affect the hospital's market share and the cost effectiveness of care.

The hospital's culture was conservative, and the institution was noted for recognizing the effects of change on an organization.

Therefore, a conservative approach to modifying the organization structure was preferred. The phrase "evolution versus revolution" was frequently used. The administrative team agreed that, sometime in the future, substantial modifications to the existing organization structure might be necessary to allow the organization to thrive and prosper. However, Ms. Glenham recommended and others concurred that there was no identified need to make changes beyond those that were seen as absolutely necessary.

The administrative team was concerned about the introduction of the change and, most specifically, what to call it. Even though many health care institutions were eagerly implementing various approaches using the industrial terminology, Mr. Tracy had serious concerns about using the word *product* in health care. Thus, the administrative team decided to refer to the effort as "service line management."

Four service lines were chosen to be initiated in the first year. Each one was seen by the administrative team as either a major current strength of the organization or a potential strength, given time and energy for development.

Orthopedics, an area of current strength, was named a service line. As a specialty service, orthopedics' strength stemmed from its large number of highly competent and subspecialized orthopedic surgeons and the commitment that the hospital had made to promote the practices of these physicians. The service area for orthopedics already was far greater than for that of most of Waller's other services.

Women's health had a history of strength and the potential to become stronger. Waller had been the first hospital in the area to develop a family-centered maternity service, and for many years had boasted the largest number of births in the state. However, other communities had developed their maternity services to a point where they were competitive with the Waller program, and thus market share had begun to drop. Also, there was evidence that women made most of the health care decisions for their families, and it was important to understand their needs and perceptions.

Occupational health was a relatively new service offered by the hospital, but was seen as a critical one to develop and expand, partly because industry had begun to look at preventive measures for maintaining a healthy work force. Workers injured on the job were contributing to higher costs. Many employers perceived wellness in terms of cost effectiveness and were willing to invest in it for their work forces. Occupational health services were offered by a number of departments throughout the hospital, including the emergency department, occupational therapy, and physical therapy, and there was a great need for integration of efforts. Economies of scale in terms of program development, promotion, and sales could be achieved through coordination. Yet, since the various departments also provided services other than occupational health, the centralization of staff members who provided that specific care into one department seemed to have more negative implications than positive. Thus, a highly coordinated effort without any radical restructuring was proposed for the occupational health service line to do joint problem solving, planning, program development, and promotion.

The cardiovascular service line was the last of the four to be developed. This service was compared to a diamond in the rough. With effective coordination, increased physician referrals, and heightened consumer awareness of the available cardiovascular resources at the facility, it was believed that this service could expand tremendously. The numbers and types of medical specialties involved in the provision of cardiovascular services was broad, which had made it difficult for the service as a whole to develop in a consistent and coordinated fashion. Duplication of equipment and services had resulted from the historical lack of coordination among the providers.

Department of Project Development Services

Historically, Waller had been an assertive and progressive institution. In the mid 1980s, management realized that the hospital's number of active projects was large and oftentimes overwhelming. Additionally, those responsible for project management sometimes did not have the skills, the time, or the resources required to effectively coordinate it. Often no one knew who was truly responsible for a project, and progress was halted by confusion and ambiguity.

Additionally, the administrative team had no good method of tracking current projects.

Thus, the Department of Project Development Services was born, and a project management process was developed by the institution. Depending upon the size of a project, the process required that it go through a number of steps, from conceptual design to evaluation. At each step senior management decided whether to proceed. Each project was assigned to a project manager, who was typically already managing the functional area most directly affected by the project, or who was ultimately responsible for the end result of the project, whether it be a program, service, or event. Depending on the size and duration of the project, a staff person from Project Development Services also could be assigned to actively support the project manager.

Frequently, a number of departments would need to be represented on a given project, so temporary workgroups were established. Each member of a workgroup was expected to be responsible for his or her department's contribution to the project's completion. Workgroup members "reported" to the project manager for those project activities. The interdepartmental workgroups, and accountability of managers of project efforts to other managers who were most often peers, broke the ground both for a task force approach to problem solving and planning and for accountability that went beyond a manager's direct superior. Suddenly, departments were required to see other departments as their customers, whose needs they had to meet. This was reinforced through both high expectations of senior management and general peer pressure. The four years of experience with the project management process paved the way for the service line management approach. Coincidentally, Ms. Glenham was the manager responsible for coordinating the project development process, and managed the department until 1988.

Composition of Service Line Teams

Based on tradition, culture, and the identified goals of the service line management effort, the administrative team decided that each service line would be represented by a team of care providers and would serve as a forum for the service line's problem solving and

planning. Team members would be representatives from the relevant medical staff departments and hospital managers or staff from
the departments that had major involvement in the provision of
care to the service line's patients. Owing to the distribution of physicians in the medical community, both representatives from the
Roberts Clinic and independent physicians often were requested to
be part of the teams.

Managers at Waller were recognized for the credibility and
influence that they had acquired in their clinical specializations.
Congruent with the evolutionary approach to the effort, the administrative team agreed that managers whose existing responsibilities
related to particular service lines could immediately be influential.
The team also felt that, at least initially, most of the service lines
did not require full-time service line management positions. Thus,
based on their level of influence as developed from clinical and
managerial competence, service line managers were identified.

The service line manager identified for orthopedics, Susan
Sailler, R.N., was the head nurse for the orthopedics floor. Judy
Starrz, M.S.N., assistant vice president of maternal and child health,
was chosen to be the service line manager for women's health.
Donna Cruisean, R.N., M.B.A., the one full-time service line manager, was promoted from head nurse for ambulatory services to
service line manager for occupational health. Mary Gerber, M.S.N.,
maintained a half-time clinical nurse specialist position for cardiac
and critical care while taking on the part-time cardiovascular service line manager position. Service line managers were paid an
additional $250 each month in a separate check.

To develop influential teams and to signal the importance of
the service line effort, a member of the administrative team was
assigned to each service line team. This position was termed the
"administrative representative," and individuals were chosen for
their interest in the particular service lines. In some areas, the administrative representative had direct involvement with previous
activities of the service or specialty. For example, Rich Fox, vice
president for clinical services, was named to the cardiovascular service line. The departments of cardiology and radiology were in Mr.
Fox's division, and thus he had direct influence over those areas. In
contrast, Carol Tanner, vice president for information services, had

no direct authority over any departments that would be represented on the women's health service line team, but she had a strong interest in the area. Jean March, vice president for nursing, was assigned to the orthopedic service line. Mr. Tracy had an intense interest in seeing the occupational health service grow and appointed himself as the administrative representative to that service line.

Service Line Reporting Relationships

Initially, service line managers reported to the administrative representative on their service lines. They also continued to report to their functional department managers for their other responsibilities. Thus, dual reporting relationships were developed. For example, the women's health service line manager, who also was the assistant vice president for maternal and child health, reported to Ms. March for nursing activities and to Ms. Tanner for service line activities. Ms. Glenham participated in each service line as a consultant to all the service line managers.

After one and one half years with this reporting structure, Ms. Glenham was promoted to the position of assistant to the president and to the administrative team. She was given broader organizational responsibilities, which included direct responsibility for the service line teams. Thus, the service line managers shifted their reporting relationship from the other administrative representatives to Ms. Glenham. For purposes of consistency, and based on the administrative representatives' interests, the other administrative team members remained a part of the service line teams.

Information and Marketing Support for Service Line Teams

The departments of marketing and management information services (MIS), excited by the new service line focus, dedicated specific individuals to develop both the data base and reporting system to support the managers and their service lines. These individuals developed strong relationships with the service line mangers. It was soon recognized, especially by the MIS staff, that they had the information and assessments that could benefit the service lines, but they did not have the relationships or familiarity with the physi-

cians and other care providers to use the information effectively.
The service line managers did have the relationships and the forum
to interact with the physicians and other professional departments,
but previously they did not have access to the information and were
not as proficient in the interpretation of the clinical and financial
data.

Positive Outcomes

The positive outcomes of the service line management effort were
significant, largely owing to the service line managers, who were
persistent and energetic in leading the organization in new directions. Their role as advocates was similar to that of "disciples," as
described in Chapter Six, in that it was necessary for them to prove
to large numbers of people that this new way of dealing with problem solving and planning was worth the time and effort, and would
result in the growth, development, and enhanced quality and efficiency of their services.

Additionally, the involved medical staff members were for
the most part extremely supportive. Attendance and participation
by physicians was a problem with only one of the four service lines.
The medical staff members were willing to participate in subgroups
of the service line to focus on specific activities and to represent their
departments and serve as communication links for feedback. It was
clear to the senior and service line managers that without physician
commitment, achievements would have been minimal. Thus, it was
important to prove to skeptical physicians that achievements were
possible and that lost opportunities not only hurt the hospital but
ultimately also hurt the medical staff's ability to provide high-
quality, cost effective care. Thus, the hospital believed that the service line efforts had built-in incentives for the physicians. It was the
job of the service line managers to get the physicians to see the
opportunity that was being afforded them.

Departmental commitment and support for the service line
teams and their efforts were also seen as significant. For the most
part, departmental managers and staff were consistent and enthu-
siastic participants in the process. Some hard lessons were learned
by some of the service lines when new opportunities were assessed

the "old" way. The old way meant that people were not as willing to look at issues creatively. Instead, they focused on the immediate impact on their departments and not necessarily on the ultimate impact on the customer, whether it be the patient, the physician, or the system itself. When this sort of thing happened, however, the service team became disappointed with its inability to solve the problem. Generally, people learned from the experience, and the next time, they looked at the opportunities and problems differently and more effectively.

The third group highly responsible for the success of the service line management effort was the administrative team. Its vision and commitment to the potential and then actual achievements that could be realized by service line management was evident from day one. Service line management was the first "core strategy" for the organization's strategic plan and thus was given a high priority by this group. Its departmental responsibilities and loyalties did not interfere with the objective assessment of service line activities. Because service lines were seen to focus on customers' needs, the administrative team members interpreted their departments' roles in meeting those needs. The administrative team's and department managers' specific responsibilities in particular service lines, as well as the administrative team's high level of involvement in establishing the service line management approach, gained their commitment, energy and support for the effort.

Interdepartmental communication and coordination improved, as did communication between the hospital managers and the medical staff. Old problems were assessed and solved in new ways. Dramatic improvements in specific medical staff relationships occurred. In many areas this increased the medical staff's trust and confidence in the hospital.

Hospital managers, particularly those in nursing, began to perceive and treat physicians as customers. Initially, this perspective was difficult for some to grasp. However, with the improvement in general relations and the recognition of the importance of physicians in solving problems and setting future directions, this concept was accepted. Additionally, the service line teams provided a forum for individuals, whether medically trained or not, to get to know one another better. One of the service lines became very social, and the relaxed nature of meetings contributed to effective work relations. Because of these interactions and resulting relations, some departments began to express their disappointment in not being able to have a greater role in service line management.

The service line teams met their general objective of developing a forum for more effective problem solving and planning by service. Physicians and department managers learned that if a problem needed to be solved, they should take it to the service line. A deliberate plan in the early days of the effort was to have some quick achievements, to gain participant commitment and support. This turned into a discipline, and the service lines generally became very action oriented.

By the second year of service line management, the information system had been developed and tested, and the service line managers had developed relationships with the marketing and MIS staff. Additionally, the service line teams had focused many of their energies on the resolution, improvement, or development of new services to meet existing needs. For a variety of reasons, the service line teams' involvement in financial and marketing matters had been less aggressive. First, the hospital felt that relations among the participants of service line management had to be formed before real progress could be made on issues relating to utilization management. Second, the hospital did not want to market services that were not highly effective and efficient. The institution had been reluctant to jump into the marketing blitz, as many health care institutions had done, and especially did not want to participate in gimmicky marketing. It was known that these concerns were on the minds of the medical staff as well, who were generally skeptical of the real intentions of service line management. Additionally, medical staff concerns over the hospital's intrusion into the physicians' realm of patient care management was evident when the service line effort was introduced. Thus, the focus of service line activities was seen as evolutionary, paralleling development of the skills of the service line managers. It was important first to maximize the quality, effectiveness, and efficiency of operations by improving communication and coordination and inspiring new assessments of old problems. Positive financial implications were expected to result. Then, a harder look at utilization and at the financial picture could be taken.

When the service line teams were given the financial and marketing data, they received them with enthusiasm, seriousness, and trust. Physicians were extremely pleased to have the institution share the kind of detail that helped them to understand the financial implications of the services they provided. At the first meetings where the information was presented, participants identified a variety of activities to try to resolve problems or at least to understand them further. Some resolutions had to do with pricing of services. The teams generally considered whether the pricing strategies of yesterday were still relevant today. Other suggestions had to do with practice patterns that were affected by hospital procedures. For example, in the cardiovascular service line, the team found that the ineffective booking procedure for pacemakers extended length of stay and contributed to inefficient provision of care. Discovery that the length of stay for myocardial infarctions was also increasing resulted in a medical staff member's recommending that the physician-chaired utilization review committee conduct an audit to profile length of stay by physician.

Waller was known to be an excellent community hospital, but it was striving for recognition as the regional referral center that it actually was in the area. Thus, the service line effort allowed marketing energies to be focused on particular services to bring attention to the institution's "centers of excellence." The hospital became more aggressive in communicating to referring physicians in the region and to the general public its state-of-the-art expertise and high quality care. It commissioned its first television commercial, and succeeded in reaching a regional audience. Informational and educational journals were developed and distributed to large numbers of consumers in the region. Radio shows also were developed as another medium for bringing the clinical experts and their competency to the general public. Educational conferences for consumers of the services—both professionals and the general public— were developed by each service line to gain recognition.

Negative Outcomes

One of the difficult issues Waller Hospital faced in implementing service line teams was the reluctance of primary care physicians to support the effort, especially the large family practice contingency.

Attempts were made to include them wherever possible, but it was rare that a physician would commit the necessary time and energy to one specialty. Women's health was an exception to this, with both an internist and a family practice physician taking active roles. However, the range of services offered in women's health was broader than in the other service lines because it was based on a large market segment and not a group of patients whose diagnoses fell into a small range of categories. Over time, however, even in women's health, the family practice representative became a less frequent participant.

The service line teams had to walk a fine line between being supportive to the primary care physicians and catering to the specialists' perceived needs for patient referrals. For example, the urologists came to the women's health service line to get support for the establishment of a continence clinic. The urologists felt that the community at large did not understand the problem and was unaware of the available medical interventions. They hypothesized that patients generally did not discuss this problem with their physicians, assuming that it was "just one of the things a woman must bear." Additionally, the urologists felt that the primary care physicians did not always investigate the needs of patients in this area and therefore did not promote the various interventions.

Thus, the urologists felt that a clinic would be an effective way to heighten access to state-of-the-art care and awareness. However, the primary care physicians expressed concern that this approach would result in patients' losing the comprehensive approach to care that they provided. This resistance led the urologists to take a less aggressive route and to plan a series of educational programs for the medical staff, as well as articles and educational events to heighten community awareness. It was hoped that in the future the clinic approach would be more accepted by the primary care contingency and then could be developed.

Clearly, the team approach meant more meetings for many people, but the participation was felt to be necessary to achieve integration. Many departments, primarily nursing and some of the therapy departments, had representation on most if not all service line teams. At first the commitment was seen as somewhat overwhelming, but as outcomes were achieved and the investment of time proved valuable, these concerns waned. Most people felt that the investment of time and energy was well worthwhile. Additionally, managers looked for opportunities to involve staff in different ways, either as service line team representatives or in new roles and responsibilities back in the department, easing the load for the manager.

Owing to the structure chosen and reporting relationships that ensued, some operational managers were "caught in the middle." For example, the head nurse for the orthopedic unit became the service line manager for the orthopedic service line. Her line manager was the assistant vice president of medical/surgical nursing. However, the service line manager's superior for service line activities initially was the vice president of nursing. This lead to some concern over lack of involvement and loss of control by the assistant vice president. When the service line managers began reporting directly to the assistant to the president, this type of tension was eased.

Whenever possible, when projects of the service line teams affected operations, the operational managers became heavily involved. For example, an opportunity assessed by the cardiovascular service line led to consideration of admitting all cardiovascular inpatients onto one patient care unit. Immediately, a subgroup was developed that included other operational managers from nursing. Ms. Glenham originally coordinated the meetings, but as soon as possible she suggested that the vice president for nursing become the effort's project manager. Eventually, when the project went from an idea to the reality of a hospitalwide realignment of inpatient units, Ms. Glenham and all but one of the service line managers were no longer needed in the workgroup.

Even with the changes in reporting relationships and the involvement of operational managers, the service line managers felt some ambiguity with their dual reporting relationships, as in some cases it was unclear what should be taken to which manager. Clearly, some of the activities identified in the service lines affected or were dependent on operational areas making changes. Thus, often the service line managers felt the need to keep both of their managers involved and aware. They also often felt this to be time consuming and confusing.

Mr. Tracy's Question

Given the accomplishments of the service line effort and the general support of the institution, Mr. Tracy wondered whether to use service line management to support other programs and services. The hospital initially chose four service lines. Two others were expected to be developed, based on the significance of the areas. However, there remained a large number of programs and services that needed an integrative management focus. The services did not necessarily need the dedicated management energy and other resources that were committed to the service lines, but they could benefit from attention. Mr. Tracy recognized this need and wondered whether less formal mechanisms to support problem solving and planning in the smaller program and service areas would work. If he did continue and extend the effort, Mr. Tracy wondered what changes he should make.

Case Analysis

Although our purpose in including the Waller Hospital case was to demonstrate implementation of change, this analysis also will touch upon structure, selection of integrative managers, and rewards. Waller's approach represents an effective fit between its strategic orientation and structure, as well as effective management of an evolutionary change process. Although Waller faced a major challenge to gaining physician involvement in the change process, the effort was largely successful. Keys to success were the evolutionary approach, development of a track record of success and proven worth of the effort on which Waller could build subsequent efforts, consistent unified support of senior management, appointment of respected clinical managers to positions as integrative managers, active management of the process of change, and sensitivity to concerns of physicians and others. Although Waller's efforts were not entirely without difficulties, they achieved substantial accomplishments and, overall, exemplify a major success.

Strategy and Structure

Waller's choice of a team structure was consistent with its evolving strategic orientation. Waller initially focused on service delivery and planning and marketing and was beginning to address budget and control issues. Since service delivery was central to Waller's approach, the choice of the team structure was appropriate and necessary to achieve the required involvement of clinicians and administrators, as discussed in Chapters Two and Seven. Teams were comprised of representatives from the various departments and medical specialties involved in providing care to patients associated with each service line.

The team structure did result in service line managers' sometimes feeling caught in the middle. This is inherent in the structural arrangements of dual accountability. Rather than deny the inherent conflict, Waller senior management acknowledged it. This allowed them to legitimize the feelings of conflict and to handle specific issues on their own merits, rather than diverting their efforts into denial of the actual conflict. The structural change that placed Ms. Glenham in the position of assistant to the president, with direct responsibility for the service line teams, was an appropriate one for reducing ambiguity in the reporting relationships. Having Ms. Glenham report directly to Mr. Tracy also reinforced the importance of the service line effort. Similarly, the administrative team's direct involvement in the service line teams demonstrated administrators' commitment and the importance of the effort. Although such participation presents a situation in which formal lines of authority are crossed, its benefits often outweigh that disadvantage, as demonstrated at Waller. However, it is important to note that in organizations that do not have the high level of trust in senior management that existed at Waller, the ambiguous reporting relationships may be problematic. This reflects the importance of considering no one element of management and organization independently.

With the establishment of dual reporting relationships, Waller's team structure began to approach a matrix structure (number 7 on the organizational continuum). It was not formally a matrix in that it did not have all of the matrix characteristics, as described in Chapter Two. For example, service line management had not yet been established as a viable career path, and budgeting and personnel decisions were not made by service line managers. The service line managers, by design, did have substantial influence over members of their teams, which is characteristic of a matrix. Thus, in addition to its advantages, Waller was experiencing, in the dual reporting relationships, some of the disadvantages characteristic of matrix structures.

Selection of Integrative Managers

The selection of service line managers was consistent with the change strategy. Service line managers had earned their credibility from their clinical constituencies, which contributed to their effectiveness at operational problem solving. As the organization's information system was developed, the service line managers were exposed to new marketing and financial information and were given support in analyzing it. Thus, their skills developed as the teams developed, and they were able to include business issues in their efforts. Ultimately, the teams were exposed to the marketing and financial data without undermining the credibility of the integrative managers.

Rewards

Senior management clearly advocated and informally rewarded behaviors that supported the service line approach, and established and supported the positions of service line managers. Significant in this effort was the direct participation of senior managers in the service line teams. Their actions spoke more loudly than words. Although the involvement of senior management created some of its own ambiguity, as noted earlier in the discussion of structure, its positive effects contrast sharply with the situations in Biscayne Hospital (Chapter Eight) and Philadelphia Hospital Medical Center (Chapter Nine).

To a limited extent, such as through Ms. Glenham's promotion, Waller has formally rewarded service line efforts. In addition, the $250 monthly salary increment symbolized the positive value the hospital placed on the service line manager role. Paying this increment in a separate check gave it even more significance. Although the formal reward system has not been used as much as it could be, senior management has clearly indicated what kinds of behaviors are desired, and additional reliance on formal rewards does not appear necessary. A more direct linkage of rewards, such as salary increases and promotions, to goal achievement could violate Waller's culture, which values relationships highly. At a later date, Waller management may need to reconsider whether to reinforce the service line effort more, through formal rewards. In the interim, there is no need to risk the unintended negative consequences of narrowly focusing behaviors through use of formal rewards, given that the desired outcomes are being achieved.

Information System

Although the case contains limited discussion of Waller's information system, it does mention availability of utilization information reported by service line and by physician. Waller has the organizational capacity to use more sophisticated financial and marketing information. Where Waller has provided teams with data on length of stay, the team members have acted to use the information effectively. Waller's emphasis on the effectiveness and efficiency of care delivery can be advanced by making more clinical and financial information available to clinicians and service line managers and their teams. Because it has established an organization structure and processes that can use the information effectively, Waller can benefit from additional development and refinement of its information system.

The Change Process

The team approach was built on the prior project management effort, in which peers were responsible to peers for the achievement of specific project-related tasks. The highly participative, work-group oriented method was already ingrained in the culture of the organization. By building on the success of its project management efforts, and then on the initial success of the new service line management effort, Waller management cultivated a positive image of the service line efforts. By achieving some initial operational successes of importance to participants in the service line teams, the evolutionary approach set a foundation for further change. Initial successes helped to transform potential passive resistance and non-commitment into support and participation, as physicians and others saw the benefits to themselves. Given the strategy of starting with small, achievable successes, it was appropriate that Waller initially did not focus on more sensitive issues, such as utilization management. As the teams developed and proved their effectiveness, and as relationships developed among team participants, the groundwork was set to face the tougher issues. Although Waller had the advantage of prior successes with project management, other institutions starting an integrative management approach without a similar history should note the importance of building a foundation of success for the new effort and not beginning with sensitive issues that initially have a small chance of being successfully changed.

The involvement and commitment of the senior management team was important for others in the institution to recognize the relative significance of the effort. Since much ambiguity exists during a major organizational change, and people in an organization look to see "which way the wind is blowing" relative to the espoused change, consistent senior management support is critical. At Waller, physicians' and department managers' participation was encouraged through senior managers' support. Additionally, senior management support was important for the empowerment of the chosen service line managers.

The hospital recognized the importance of physician involvement and acted to achieve physician interest, involvement, and eventual support of the process. Early in the evolutionary approach to change, it was the service line managers' responsibility to prove to their physician members, as well as to department manager participants, that this new problem solving and planning effort was worth their investment of time and effort. This is especially difficult to achieve in a community hospital, where physicians' time commitments to meetings directly reduce their time to see patients and derive income. The hospital's choice of terminology was significant in reflecting that the new approach would not reduce patient focus. In fact, by focusing on patient care issues, the service line implementation effort addressed the one subject that all participants felt was important to them.

Given the distinct factions in the medical staff, it was important to include representatives from both the Roberts Clinic and the independent physician group. Had it not included both factions, Waller would have risked further splintering of the medical staff and accusations of favoring one group or the other. Since both physician groups were important to Waller's continued success and Waller had to be responsive to both, it needed input and involvement from both. Maintaining a focus on patient care, in contrast to issues of control or turf, helped in dealing with potentially competing perspectives.

Waller managers learned that primary care physicians and specialists had differing perceptions of what was needed for their patients. The specialists, for example, often envisioned specialty clinics, such as the continence clinic, which the primary care physicians resisted. They instead agreed to participate in a more educationally oriented approach for the general public, for specific patient groups, or for themselves. It is important to note that the training, concerns, and economic incentives are different for the specialists and the primary care physicians. Since integrative efforts, as exemplified by Waller, affect the different groups and provide opportunities for the groups to express their views, management may hear of some of the differences in perspectives and interests for the first time through the integrative efforts. Hospital management should not be surprised by these differences; they have existed for a long time. Sensitivity in dealing with the differences and the ability to see others' positions and negotiate effectively were key to success of the integrative efforts.

Because Waller's approach was consistent with its somewhat conservative culture, resistance to the change effort was minimal. The approach did not present a shock to the organization that could have provided a rallying point for organizing resistance to change. Mr. Tracy and the administrative team communicated a vision focused on developing high-quality programs and services that would ensure the cost effectiveness of care. They said and confirmed through their actions that gimmicky marketing efforts would not be pursued. Rather, they said they would promote only high-quality services. This helped to alleviate physician fears that "service line management" meant "gimmicky marketing." With this barrier reduced, additional physician acceptance was achieved.

The effort at Waller Hospital resulted in improved relations, communication, and coordination between the hospital and physicians, among hospital departments, and, in some areas, between the hospital and the community. Additionally, the effort brought together various medical specialties and, in some cases, competing physician groups. Senior management and integrative managers demonstrated increased awareness of the medical staff's concerns and worked to develop positive relationships with them.

By the end of the case, people at Waller who have not been involved in the service line effort have indicated that they too wish to be part of service line teams. This is a strong indication of the success of establishing integrative management as the way of solving problems at Waller. As powerful as the integrative approach is for addressing problems that cross departmental and medical specialty lines, however, it also is expensive in terms of the time and effort of participants. It is essential that the team approach not be applied blindly throughout the hospital. Rather, for issues that are not of a continuing nature, it is more appropriate to use the less permanent approach of task forces, or to appoint integrative managers who can coordinate efforts through direct contact with the involved departments and physicians. This is consistent with Waller's project management efforts. It does not conflict with the team approach, and it allows the appropriate structural arrangements to be used to address varying organizational needs.

Overall, the Waller case demonstrates an integration of appropriate decisions with regard to organization structure, selection of integrative managers, and reward and information systems, as well as an effective orchestration and management of an evolutionary change process. It has built on its strengths and, through consistent senior management support, clearly indicated the direction for others in the organization to follow. Although at the beginning of their change efforts many organizations do not have the strong relationships and organizational culture present at Waller, the case demonstrates a change process that provides examples and guidance to others.

Chapter Fourteen

Using Organization Design to Facilitate Innovation

Initially through development of concepts, and then through case examples and analyses, this book has presented a framework for developing innovative organizations that are responsive to customers, that empower staff, and that are effective in delivery of care. Given the different experiences described in the cases, it should be clear that building an effective organization is more than recruiting good people. In addition, no single element of the framework is sufficient to achieve these desired outcomes. The elements interact with each other and must be managed as a system.

Central to the framework is the structure of the organization. Decisions about how to organize have profound implications on hospitals and other organizations. Until very recently, most hospitals have not used organization design to their advantage. Many people have discounted the importance of organization structure because they have considered it to be nothing more than boxes and lines on a piece of paper. These boxes and lines are but a crude way to symbolize relationships among people, distribution of power, control over resources, and locus of decision making. These are real things that come to life through people's behavior. Structure also has a major impact on how people perceive what is important and how to get things done in their organization. Hospitals must move beyond the state where some people work extraordinarily hard to get things done in spite of the organization structure, others get some things done but inefficiently or ineffectively, and still others simply do not get things done. Hospital leaders must use the structure to facilitate rather than hinder their employees' efforts.

Some hospitals have altered their structures, reporting relationships, and systems, but have done so in a hit-or-miss fashion, without the guidance of a roadmap to organization design. The preceding chapters have provided a roadmap, in terms of concepts and case examples. In using the roadmap, managers must recognize that—contrary to what is promoted by zealous advocates of one type of structure or system or another—each organizational form has inherent advantages and disadvantages. These must be considered relative to the strategy and organizational needs of a given hospital, and structure, rewards, information system, selection of integrative managers, and the change process must be used together to achieve the desired results.

In Bayview Medical Center and Waller Memorial Hospital, these elements were integrated well, and, on balance, those hospitals were reaping far more benefits than disadvantages from their organizational arrangements. In Philadelphia Hospital Medical Center, Biscayne Hospital, and Hillside Health Services, senior managers seem to have lost the roadmap. Their decision making does not appear to be guided by concepts that could allow them to avoid costly errors. Hanna-Thorndike Hospital reaped substantial benefits, but was also experiencing many disadvantages from its innovative arrangements. With a better roadmap, it could have chosen a structure, reward system, and information system that provided better balance between benefits and dysfunctional outcomes.

One thing that is consistently clear across the case studies is the importance of senior management's support for an organizational innovation. That support was evident at Bayview Medical Center, Hanna-Thorndike Hospital, and Waller Memorial Hospital. It was not evident at Biscayne Hospital or Philadelphia Hospital Medical Center, and it was inconsistent at Hilltop Health Services. The differences in results are dramatic.

Although roadmaps are static, organizations are not. Managers must consider both the immediate and long-term effects of their organizational choices. Short-term benefits of an approach may have long-term liabilities. For example, the initial operational advantages of a program organization are outweighed in the long term by the negative impact on maintaining state-of-the-art professional competence and standards. However, some short-term negative aspects of a change can be addressed over a period of time. For example, the pain associated with change can be replaced with satisfaction gained through a successfully functioning organization.

Most hospitals have focused on the individual disciplines and functions to the extent that for some the hospital exists more for the disciplines than for the patients. This is why many people chuckle but accept the metaphor of a hospital as a number of independent fiefdoms connected by a common heating system. Because the patient is not just "a hip," "a heart," or any other single organ system or body part and cannot be cared for by any single discipline, hospitals must develop more effective ways to integrate. This is why this book has focused on organizational integration.

Managing integration in hospitals cannot be left to chance. The organization structure and other systems must be used to facilitate integration in management and in clinical work. This will reduce fragmentation and allow professionals more opportunities to gain satisfaction from their work by addressing patient needs more effectively.

This book has addressed product line management and its variations, both in a chapter and through the cases. The topic was included not because we espouse product line management, but because it is one of the few approaches to organizational integration in health care that has had some positive outcomes. It also has not worked in many situations, as illustrated through several of the cases, which we believe show the process in vivo, as it were. Many of the concepts can be applied without the negative implications of putting business objectives before patient care. History has shown that, in the long run, market success depends on the ability to deliver a quality product or service.

Beyond the concepts presented in this book, there are several other innovations that are occurring in hospitals. Primary among these are total quality management, case management, and role restructuring. The focus on organization structure, rewards, information systems, and the change process is philosophically congruent and complementary with these other approaches. Each of these areas has a literature of its own, whereas hospital leaders lack an effective roadmap to organization design and integration. Quite clearly, much empirical research needs to be done to prove or disprove the concepts discussed in this book. We encourage that work. However, we hope to have provided examples of and insights into the best thinking about how to implement innovative, integrative approaches in health care.

The 1990s are a time for change in health care. Payment reform, changing philosophies of practice, and closer relationships with and participation by physicians are well on their way. Even more radical change is likely to come to address issues of cost, access, and quality. To address these challenges, not only must national policy and payment mechanisms change, but also institutions that provide care must change. The challenges are enormous, but so are the opportunities. Many of the paradigms that govern how hospitals function need to be set aside and new approaches taken. To do this requires creating a climate in hospitals that promotes creativity and guided risk taking. It is a time of opportunity for innovation in structure, information systems, and management practices. In fact, innovation is a necessity.

No single approach is sufficient to bring about all of the changes needed in health care organizations. This book does not pretend to provide a quick fix or even a simple fix. A multifaceted approach to organization change is needed to meet the challenges of the 1990s and beyond. Those leaders who recognize the complexity of health care organizations, who have the vision to empower their staff and employees, who have sound management concepts to guide them, and who are able to work with ambiguity, rather than deny its existence, will have the greatest success. Changes in health care are too complex to be accomplished by individuals working alone. Integrative efforts are essential to meet the challenges ahead.

References

Ackoff, R. L. *The Art of Problem Solving*. New York: Wiley, 1978.

Alfireric, J., Kroman, B., and Ruflin, P. "Informational Needs for a Product Line Management System." *Healthcare Financial Management*, 1987, *41*(3), 60–65.

Anderson, R. A. "Products and Product-line Management in Nursing." *Nursing Administration Quarterly*, 1985, *10*(1), 65–72.

Arrildt, W. D. "Adapting Organizational Structure to a Changing Environment." *Radiology Management*, 1986, 22–25.

Batchelor, G. J., Butler, P. W., and Jellinek, L. A. "Clinical Profiles Manage Quality, Cost of Hospital Product." *Healthcare Financial Management*, 1987, *41*(7), 66–72.

Bauer, P. S., and Rinaldo, J. A. "The Case Mix System," from Arthur Andersen and Co., and Providence Hospital, Southfield, Michigan. Presented at the 1st annual conference of the American Association for Medical Systems and Informatics, October 1982, 55–63.

Bennett, J. P. "Standard Cost Systems Lead to Efficiency and Profitability." *Healthcare Financial Management*, 1985, *39*(9), 46–54.

Bird, G. A. "Product-line Management and Nursing." *Nursing Management,* 1988, *19*(5), 46–48.

Blau, P. M. *The Dynamics of Bureaucracy.* Chicago: University of Chicago Press, 1955.

Boshard, N. "A Planning and Marketing Prototype for Changing Health Care Organizations." *Health Care Strategic Management,* 1986, *4*(11), 14–18.

Burns, L. R. "Matrix Management in Hospitals: Testing Theories of Matrix Structure and Development." *Administrative Science Quarterly,* 1989, *34,* 349–368.

Charns, M. P. "Breaking the Tradition Barrier: Managing Integration in Health Care Facilities." *Health Care Management Review,* 1976, *1*(1), 55–67.

Charns, M. P. "Product Line Management and Clinical Costing Systems." *Australian Health Review,* 1986, *41*(3), 60–66.

Charns, M. P., Lawrence, P. R., and Weisbord, M. R. "Organizing Multiple Function Professionals in Academic Medical Centers." *Management Science* (special issue on prescriptive models of organization), 1977, *5,* 71–88.

Charns, M. P., and Schaefer, M. J. *Health Care Organizations: A Model for Management.* Englewood Cliffs, N.J.: Prentice-Hall, 1983.

Charns, M. P., and Smith, L. J. "Product Line Management and Continuum of Care." *Health Matrix,* 1989, *VII*(1), 40–49.

Cleverly, W. O. "Product Costing for Health Care Firms." *Health Care Management Review,* 1987, *12*(4), 39–48.

Cole, G., and Brown, C. "Product-line Management: Concept to Reality." *Topics in Health Care Finance,* 1988, *14*(3), 62–75.

Cooper, J. C., and Surer, J. D. "Product Line Cost Estimation: A Standard Cost Approach." *Healthcare Financial Management,* 1988, *42*(4), 60–70.

Davis, S. M., and Lawrence, P. R. *Matrix.* Reading, Mass.: Addison-Wesley, 1977.

Deal, T. E., and Kennedy, A. A. *Corporate Cultures.* Reading, Mass.: Addison-Wesley, 1982.

Delbecq, A. L., Van de Ven, A. H., and Gustafson, D. H. *Group Techniques for Program Planning: A Guide to Nominal Group and Delphi Processes.* Glenville, Ill.: Scott, Foresman, 1975.

Dominguez, G. S. *Product Management*. New York: American Management Association, 1971.

Dumbaugh, K., and Demarzi-Jeye, D. "Choose Your Weapon: Picking a Product Line Management System That Produces." *Software in Healthcare*, 1987, *5*(2), 32–37.

Fackelmann, K. A. "Cleveland Hospital on the Road to Product Line Management." *Modern Healthcare*, 1985, *15*(24), 70–77.

Fetter, R. B., and Freeman, J. L. "Diagnosis-Related Groups: Product Line Management Within Hospitals." *Academic Management Review*, 1983, *11*(1), 41–54.

Folger, J. C., and Gee, E. P. *Product Management for Hospitals: Organizing for Profitability*. Chicago: American Publishing, 1987.

Fottler, M. D. "Health Care Organizational Performance: Present and Future Research." *Journal of Management*, 1987, *13*(2), 367–391.

Fottler, M. D., and Repasky, L. J. "Attitudes of Hospital Executives Toward Product Line Management: A Pilot Survey." *Health Care Management Review*, 1988, *13*(3), 15–22.

Frommelt, J. J., Scheuerman, J. L., and Fillmore, J. H. "Finance and Marketing: Birth of a Profitable Relationship." *Healthcare Financial Management*, 1987, 25–32.

Galbraith, J. R. *Designing Complex Organizations*. Reading, Mass.: Addison-Wesley, 1973.

Go, R., and Gregg, R. H. "Strategic Planning and Product Line Management Under DRG-Based Prospective Payment." *DRG Monitor*, 1985, *2*(6), 1–8.

Goodrich, R. G., and Hastings, G. R. "St. Luke's Hospital Reaps Benefits by Using Product Line Management." *Modern Healthcare*, 1985, *15*(4), 157–158.

Gray, R. J. "Marketing for Success through Product-line Management." *Topics in Health Care Finance*, 1988, *14*(3), 76–83.

Hackman, J. R., and Oldham, G. "Development of the Job Diagnostic Survey." *Journal of Applied Psychology*, 1975, 159–170.

Harmon, R. G., and Kirkman-Liff, B. L. "Matrix/Team Management in a Public Health Department." *Journal of Ambulatory Care Management*, 1984, *7*(2), 1–12.

Hoffman, B. "Product Line Management: Streamlining Service,

Management, and Staff Performance." *Osteopathic Hospital Leadership,* 1986, *30*(5), 5, 20.

Jacobs, P., and Szafran, A. J. "Establish Transfer Prices in a Product Line Setting." *Healthcare Financial Management,* 1987, *41*(11), 86–88.

Johnson, J. E., Arvidson, A. C., Costa, L. L., Hekhuis, F. M., Lennox, L. A., Marshall, S. B., and Moran, M. J. "Marketing Your Nursing Product Line: Reaping the Benefits." *Journal of Nursing Administration,* 1987, *17*(11), 29–33.

Kerr, S. "On the Folly of Rewarding 'A' While Hoping for 'B.' " *Academy of Management Journal,* 1975, *18*(4), 769–783.

Lawrence, P. R., and Lorsch, J. W. *Organization and Environment: Managing Differentiation and Integration.* Boston: Division of Research, Harvard Business School, 1967.

Lawrence, P. R., and Lorsch, J. W. "New Management Job: The Integrator." *Harvard Business Review,* 1968, *45*(6), 142–151.

Leatt, P., Shortell, S. M., and Kimberly, J. R. "Organization Design." In S. M. Shortell and A. D. Kaluzny, *Health Care Management: A Text in Organizational Theory and Behavior.* (2nd ed.) New York: Wiley, 1988.

Lewin, K. "Group Decision and Social Change." In T. M. Newcomb and E. L. Hartley (eds.), *Readings in Social Psychology.* New York: Holt, Rinehart & Winston, 1958.

Linden, R. "Materials Management's Role in Product Line Development." *Hospital Materials Management,* 1986, *11*(6), 8–12.

Lowe, L. "How to Avoid Chaos in the Transition to Product Line Management." *Health Care Strategic Management,* 1987, *5*(4), 9–13.

Lutz, S. "Hospitals Consider Product Line Management Techniques to Better Meet Customer Needs." *Modern Healthcare,* 1987, *17*(8), 70–74.

McDaniel, R. R., Thomas, J. B., Ashmos, D. P., and Smith, J. P. "The Use of Decision Analysis for Organizational Design: Reorganizing a Community Hospital." *Journal of Applied Behavioral Science,* 1987, *23*(3), 337–350.

MacStravic, R. S. "Product Line Administration in Hospitals." *Health Care Management Review,* 1986, *11*(2), 35–43.

Manning, M. F. "Product Line Management: Will It Work in

Health Care?" *Healthcare Financial Management*, 1987, *41*(1), 23-32.

Nackel, J. G. "Competitive Advantage Through Organizational Structure." *Healthcare Executive*, 1988, *3*(3), 15-17.

Nackel, J. G., Fenaroli, P. J., and Kis, G. "Product-line Performance Reporting: A Key to Cost Management." *Healthcare Financial Management*, 1987, *41*(11), 54-58.

Nackel, J. G., and Kues, I. W. "Product-line Management: Systems and Strategies." *Hospital and Health Services Administration*, 1986, *31*(2), 109-123.

Neuhauser, D. "The Hospital as a Matrix Organization." *Hospital Administration*, 1972, *17*(4), 8-25.

Patterson, D. J., and Thompson, K. A. "Product Line Management: Organization Makes the Difference." *Healthcare Financial Management*, 1987, *41*(2), 66-72.

Perlman, D., and Takacs, G. J. "The 10 Stages of Change." *Nursing Management*, 1990, *21*(4), 33-38.

Porn, L. and Manning, M. "Strategic Pricing: Hitting the Mark with Pricing Strategies." *Healthcare Financial Management*, 1988, *42*(1), 27-32.

Rice, A. J. "PLM in Action." *Healthcare Forum*, 1987, *30*(1), 29-32.

Rice, W. W. "Oncology and Product Line Management: Pitfalls in Practice." *Health Care Strategic Management*, 1986, *4*(10), 4-8.

Rosenberg, V. L. "The Myth of Reimbursement-Controlled Purchasing." In H. Brehm and R. Mullner (eds.), *Health Care Technology and the Competitive Environment*. New York: Praeger, 1989, 91-104.

Ruffner, J. K. "Product Line Management: How Six Healthcare Institutions Make It Work." *Healthcare Forum*, 1986, *29*(5), 11-14.

Sabatino, F. G., and Grayson, M. A. "Diversification: More Black Ink Than Red Ink." *Hospitals*, 1988, *62*(1), 36-42.

Salter, V. "Product Line Management: Its Meaning and Future Promise." *Health Care Strategic Management*, 1986, *4*(5), 13-15.

Saxe, J. G. "The Blind Men and the Elephant." In *The Illustrated Treasury for Children*. New York: Grosset & Dunlap, 1970.

Senge, P. M. *The Fifth Discipline: The Art and Practice of the Learning Organization.* New York: Doubleday, 1990a.

Senge, P. M. "The Leader's New Work: Building Learning Organizations." *Sloan Management Review*, 1990b, *32*(1), 7–23.

Siegrist, R. B., and Blish, C. S. "Cost Accounting, Management Control, and Planning in Health Care." *American Journal of Hospital Pharmacy*, 1988, *45*, 372–379.

Smith, T., Leatt, P., Ellis, P., and Fried, B. "Decentralized Hospital Management: Rationale, Potential, and Two Case Examples." *Health Matrix*, 1989, *VII*(1), 11–17.

Souhrada, L. "Neuroscience: Your Next Center of Excellence?" *Hospitals*, 1988, *62*(4), 88.

Stoelwinder, J. U., and Charns, M. P. "A Task Field Model of Organization Analysis and Design." *Human Relations*, 1981, *34*(9), 743–762.

Stoelwinder, J. U., and Clayton, P. S. "Hospital Organization Development: Changing the Focus from 'Better Management' to 'Better Patient Care.' " *Journal of Applied Behavioral Science*, 1978, *14*(3), 400–414.

Super, K. E. "Product Line Management Needs Careful Implementation." *Modern Healthcare*, 1987, *17*(10), 99.

Thompson, J. D. *Organizations in Action.* New York: McGraw-Hill, 1967.

Toohey, E. M., Shillinger, F. L., and Baranowski, S. L. "Planning Alternative Delivery Systems: An Organizational Assessment." *Journal of Nursing Administration*, 1985, *15*(12), 9–15.

Touche Ross Survey Results, *Hospitals*, May 20, 1987, p. 56.

Tucker, S., and Burr, R. M. "Strategic Market Planning." *Topics in Health Care Finance*, 1988, *14*(3), 44–55.

Weisbord, M. R. "Why Organization Development Hasn't Worked (So Far) in Medical Centers." *Health Care Management Review*, 1976, *1*(2), 17–28.

Weisbord, M. R. *Productive Workplaces: Organizing and Managing for Dignity, Meaning, and Community.* San Francisco: Jossey-Bass, 1987.

Weisbord, M. R., Stoelwinder, J. U., and Pava, C.H.P. "Involving Physicians in Hospital Cost Containment: Developing an Action

Research Strategy." *Journal of Health and Human Resource Administration,* 1983, *6*(1), 23–45.

Wodinsky, H. B., Egan, D., and Markel, F. "Product Line Management in Oncology: A Canadian Experience." *Hospital and Health Services Administration,* 1988, *33*(2), 221–236.

Woodward, J. *Industrial Organization: Theory and Practice.* Oxford: Oxford University Press, 1965.

Yano-Fong, D. "Advantages and Disadvantages of Product-Line Management." *Nursing Management,* 1988, *19*(5), 27–31.

Index